Collaborating to Improve Community Health

Kathryn Johnson

Wynne Grossman

Anne Cassidy

EDITORS

Foreword by Tyler Norris

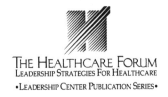

THE HEALTHCARE FORUM
LEADERSHIP STRATEGIES FOR HEALTHCARE
•LEADERSHIP CENTER PUBLICATION SERIES•

Collaborating to Improve Community Health

Workbook and Guide to Best Practices
in Creating Healthier Communities
and Populations

Jossey-Bass Publishers
San Francisco

Substantial discounts on bulk quantities of Jossey-Bass books are available to corporations, professional associations, and other organizations. For details and discount information, contact the special sales department at Jossey-Bass Inc., Publishers (415) 433-1740; Fax (800) 605-2665.

For sales outside the United States, please contact your local Simon & Schuster International Office.

Jossey-Bass Web address: http://www.josseybass.com

Manufactured in the United States of America.

Library of Congress Cataloging-in-Publication Data

Collaborating to improve community health : workbook and guide to best
    practices in creating healthier communities and populations /
    Kathryn Johnson, Wynne Grossman, and Anne Cassidy, editors.
        p.   cm.
    Includes bibliographical references
    ISBN 0-7879-1079-1
    1. Community health services. 2. Health planning. I. Johnson,
Kathryn, date. II. Grossman, Wynne, date. III. Cassidy,
Anne, date.
RA427.C59 1997
362.1'2—DC21   97–22974

PB Printing   10 9 8 7 6 5 4 3 2 1   FIRST EDITION

Contents

This workbook and guide was a multidisciplinary team effort of **The Healthcare Forum** staff, advisors and national consultants.

Project Advisors/Contributors
Best Practices Advisory Panel Members (See page xx)

The Healthcare Forum Project Staff
Kathryn Johnson, President/CEO
Wynne Grossman, Director, Research and Development
Anne Cassidy, Healthier Communities Manager
Anna Mangum, Consultant

The Healthcare Forum Staff Advisors
Keith McCandless, Director, Quality Improvement Networks
Carrie Morris, Quality Improvement Networks Manager
Susanna Trasolini, PhD, Special Projects Advisor
David Zimmerman, Research and Development Manager
Swati Fanse, Intern

Writers
Main Text: Anne Cassidy
Case Studies: Joe Flower, Writer, The Change Project

Community Editors
Micky Roberts, Clarkston Health Collaborative, Clarkston, Georgia
Barbara Strack, Growing Into Life Task Force, Aiken, South Carolina

Copyeditor
John Maybury, Consultant

Design and Production of the Contents
Allen Schlossman, President, Allen Craig Communication and Design
Jo-Anne Rosen, President, Wordrunner
Anne Cassidy
David Zimmerman

Foreword

A child is a person who is going to carry on what you started. He is going to sit where you are sitting, and when you are gone, attend to those things which you think are important. You may adopt the policies you please, but how they are carried out depends on him. He will assume control of your cities, states and nations. He is going to move in and take over your churches, schools, universities, and corporations—and the fate of humanity is in his hands.

—*Abraham Lincoln*

Growing a healthier community is a lifelong process, one that requires our constant nurturing and vigilance. Healthy communities emerge from healthy cultures. They do not come about simply because of a grant, a project, or an assessment and planning effort. These are but tools. When we work toward a healthier community by implementing such tools, we often find that any lasting positive change has more to do with the nature of the leadership and with the process employed than with the product itself. Lessons of sustained benefit in communities point to such factors as how people are meaningfully engaged, how trust and relationships are built, and how the creativity and resources of the community are mobilized toward a shared vision for the future. Leaders cannot dictate or control any of these factors; they can only provide a fertile place for them to happen. As Lincoln reminds us, for the sake of the future we must be mindful of what we stand for and what we invest in, not simply what we proclaim.

Sustaining positive change in community calls for a new form of leadership. *Community* implies common interest and shared aspiration and ownership. When leaders seek to be in front of the pack with the best idea and then work to get others to buy in, the result is often simply that they have maneuvered others into their camp. Leaders of that genre rarely build true community, despite the short-term boost to their image. This approach is too focused on the leaders themselves, not the people involved. Sadly, this leadership style has contributed to great cynicism and mistrust in our society. It has pushed ordinary citizens, who seek authenticity and substance, to the margins.

Emergent leaders in healthy communities understand that they are not the locus of change. Rather, the locus of real change is in every person, every family, every home, and every workplace, civic space and place of worship. The leader's job is therefore to help unleash the potential in every person, in each of these places. It is at this most personal level that healthy lives and communities develop. A mixed legacy of "best-laid plans" and trillions of dollars spent on programs serves as a testament to the difficulty of building community from the outside. Large-scale change begins as an internal process at home, at work, and at play. This should constantly remind us how and where to focus our energies.

There are clear roles for everyone in creating positive community change. One of the more important roles is in changing how our organizations think and how they allocate resources. These changes include influencing their visions, missions, goals, and resource allocation toward community-based solutions. In many cases, we must begin by redefining the work of our institutions.

For business and industry, building community often means starting within their own frameworks: by operating in a manner that makes a profit but that also builds the broader wealth of the people, community and environment on which they depend. For many nonprofits and related organizations, building community means moving beyond image, self-preservation, turf battles, and provision of dependency-building services. These behaviors fragment resources, create half-solutions, and sap the will and confidence of people in community. For philanthropy, building community means seeing the value in the "softer" side of community-building activity—much as we would see the raising of a child—as a long-term proposition grounded in building relationships, self-confidence and skills. This decries the one-time, short-term, "show me the outcomes in three years" philosophy that encourages communities to distort the use of their own resources in order to attract others. Although communities should be able to point convincingly to promising results along the way, the real proof may take a generation to harvest.

For healthcare, building community means reallocating resources toward the mission of creating health and well-being, not solely treating disease. It means creating partnerships with schools, churches, businesses and civic groups, and seeing the whole community as an extension of the "health system." At a minimum, building community must begin with providing basic care and preventative services for the tens of millions of uninsured. For the faith community, it means actively carrying out a physical dimension of their spiritual mission. There is no deeper way to understand our creation or to make more relevant the great teachings, than to serve. For the media, building community means educating, not simply informing. *Educating* implies framing issues in a manner that promotes understanding and action. For government, it requires no longer doing for community what it can best do for itself. It means being responsive to community realities and listening to the community for guidance in fulfilling the government's roles. These roles include serving people as a tool for social change and working to help allocate resources for the common good in a manner that engenders widespread opportunity and equity. Ultimately, building community implies a requirement of citizens to inform themselves, to accept responsibility for what's going on in their communities, and to participate actively in the process of governance.

Today, we hear the call for a deepened sense of community and for more personal responsibility: a desire both to be part of something bigger and for greater accountability. But how do community and accountability grow? Not through such activities as attacking government as the enemy, or seeing such groups as immigrants and the poor as the roots of our problems. This thinking simply frames the problem as "other," rather than "us." Building community health and quality of life must be seen as an investment by each of us in people and in society, an investment that ultimately returns benefit to the economy and us all. This is about community as a fabric, not solely a handful of strong, disconnected threads, each with a separate role.

Collaborating to Improve Community Health builds a foundation of learning from a powerful movement underway in America. It is a movement of multisectoral, comprehensive, community-based health and quality-of-life improvement initiatives that are seeking local solutions to address tough challenges. The movement has its roots in community, not in a national or organizational agenda. At its core are valuing and employing local resources for positive change. It is not about getting more but about effectively using what we have. It implies sharing tools and pooling resources in new ways. It brings together business, government, nonprofit, healthcare, faith community and citizen leaders to address community health and quality of life collaboratively. In the end, this movement's greatest contribution may be in revitalizing our democracy by more meaningfully involving citizens in the work of their community.

This "communities" movement goes by hundreds of names at the local level, but "Healthy Communities" has become one of the more popular. Part of this phenomenon is the universal appeal of health and wholeness, concepts that embrace the physical, emotional, mental and spiritual dimensions of our lives. Especially important is that a healthy community recognizes that most of what creates health has little to do with the medical care system: people's health and quality of life are dependent on many community systems and factors—not solely on access to a well-functioning medical care system. The success stories of healthy communities point to other formal and informal systems that contribute to sustained health: access to quality education, lifelong learning, and skill development; to affordable and adequate housing; to safe places for recreation and for religious and cultural expression; to jobs that inspire and pay a livable wage; to healthy ecosystems; to an honoring of diversity; and to meaningful opportunity for volunteerism and civic engagement.

We are all concerned with crime, drugs, child and domestic abuse, the decline of our inner cities and rural towns, families in crisis, lowering real wage rates and poverty, development patterns of sprawl and congestion, and more. In the face of these challenges to society, the Healthy Communities movement is an organic response. An analogy can be made with the human immune system, kicking into action in response to the presence of disease. Healthy communities build wisdom, power and resilience. Like every community, they have challenges, but they continually find creative ways to address them. They develop thinking processes, community-building skills, organizational structures and resource allocation processes relevant to their emerging realities.

Healthy communities understand power. Power involves who gets to sit at the table when policy and community decisions are made; it involves how those decisions are made and how various resources flow. Healthy communities know how to involve the diversity of their community in making decisions and how to wisely invest their resources in what creates community well-being. They have considered the future for all, not simply the short-term institutional survival of private interests. One can learn a lot about a change effort by looking at the roster of who decides what, and how the budget allocates resources.

It is becoming increasingly clear to leaders from both sides of the political aisle that if the United States is to solve its deepest, most vexing problems, the solution will be found at the local level. Around the country, leaders in business, nonprofit, government, faith, healthcare and the community are successfully mobilizing innovative partnerships that model inclusion and broad-based ownership for outcomes. And as the federal government shifts responsibility to states and communities for solutions and action, the need for communities to produce even better results is increased. The diverse skills and capacities of communities are substantial, but in too many cases they are undervalued, latent and poorly mobilized. Community leaders, and the organizations that inform and support them, must take on this added responsibility to enhance the effectiveness of all members of the community.

Identifying, evaluating and highlighting best and promising practices; sharing tools and stories; and avoiding duplication of resources—all these activities are essential as community initiatives grow across the nation. We see time and again that the real question in community is not what needs to be done but how we will do it effectively. How can we ensure that behaviors and practices are part of how people live and how organizations operate? How can we better use the various assets of the community? How can we better equip those leaders and organizations that are willing to serve as catalysts, conveners, and linkers of resources?

This book contains the combined wisdom of leaders from scores of community-based initiatives across North America. At the same time, congratulations go to The Healthcare Forum and its members, who have long worked to deepen organizational understanding of what actually creates healthier communities, and what creating healthy communities implies for leaders. The book is a celebration of learning from numerous communities across the nation. These communities have found ways to deepen the involvement of diverse community members, create a shared vision based on lasting values, build on their assets, set priorities that enhance the capacity of the community, mobilize tangible action, and measure real progress through indicators that allow continuous improvement.

At the Coalition for Healthy Cities and Communities, we are tracking hundreds of organizations and over 1,200 communities in the United States that in some form are doing "healthy community" work. In its work to directly link thousands of organizational and community efforts with each other in an environment of "peer learning," the Coalition applauds the Best Practices and tools that follow in this volume. These resources must be shared as widely and as effectively as possible for maximum benefit to America's communities. The findings in this book will encourage many thousands of citizens across the country who are working to create measurable health improvement. It can assist them in taking their local initiatives to the next level. And it can help provide credibility to local initiatives by helping skeptical community leaders see that this work is happening around the United States and is producing measurable results.

The idea of a healthy community and the approaches to help bring it about represent a new sense of hope and possibility for the United States. What has evolved over the past decade is a national network of value-laden relationships that set a tone for a new level of health and quality of life. This network has reframed the idea of *community improvement*. Community-based initiatives cannot be seen merely as projects that must appeal to limited "charity" dollars; they now rightly serve as investment advisors for what creates and sustains community health. Most important, these initiatives have begun to make a compelling case that long-term economic vitality rests on healthy people, a healthy society, a healthy ecosystem. In the end, it is these latter forms of wealth that will define the environment our children inherit and shape who they become.

May 1997

Tyler Norris
Director, Coalition for Healthy Cities and Communities
Boulder, Colorado

Community Contributors

We acknowledge the following organizations for their insight into community collaboration and countless contributions to the development of this workbook.

Advocate Health Care
Congregational Health Services
205 West Towny Avenue
Park Ridge, IL 60068
ph: (847) 698-4755
fx: (847) 692-5109
Contact: Ann Solari-Twadell
Director

African American Breast Cancer Alliance
17 South High Street
Suite 1015
Columbus, OH 43215
ph: (614) 228-2220
fx: (614) 228-2285
Contact: Marlene Miller
Corporate VP/Community Initiatives

Archbishop's Commission on Community Health
Catholic Community Service
325 North Newstead
St. Louis, MO 63108
ph: (314) 531-0511
fx: (314) 531-0511
Contact: Mary Lou Stubbs
Development Committee Chair

Asian Health Initiative
New England Medical Center
750 Washington Street, Box 017
Boston, MA 02111
ph: (617) 636-5438
fx: (617) 636-8249
Contact: Linda Chin
Associate Administrator for Planning and Marketing

Bethel New Life
4355 West Washington
Chicago, IL 60624
ph: (312) 826-5540
fx: (312) 826-5728
Contact: Marcia Turner
Public Relations Specialist

Central Oklahoma 2020
4545 North Lincoln, Suite 114
Oklahoma City, OK 73105
ph: (405) 236-0521
fx: (405) 272-0265
Contact: Deborah Redwine
Stakeholder

Chicago Department of Public Health
DePaul Center
333 South State Street, Room 2134
Chicago, IL 60604-3972
ph: (312) 747-9884
fx: (312) 747-9786
Contact: D. Patrick Lenihan
Deputy Commissioner

City of Flin Flon
Healthy Flin Flon
Box 100
Flin Flon, MB, CANADA R8A-1M6
ph: (204) 687-3190
fx: (204) 687-5829
Contact: Adele Crocker
Coordinator

Clay Organized for Wellness, Inc.
P.O. Box 120
Clay, WV 25043
ph: (304) 587-4126
fx: (304) 587-4181
Contact: Melody Reed
Coordinator

Community Council of Greater Dallas
2121 Main Street, Suite 500
Dallas, TX 75201-4383
ph: (214) 741-5851
fx: (214) 748-6051
Contact: Tracy Curts
Project Director

Community Choices 2010
404 East 15th Street, Suite 11
Greater Vancouver Chamber of Commerce
Vancouver, WA 98663
ph: (360) 694-2588
fx: (360) 693-8279
Contact: Lynne Conner
Executive Director

Community Healthcare Network
P.O. Box 790
Columbus, GA 31902-0790
ph:(706) 660-6110
fx:(706) 660-6511
Contact: Kevin Sass
Vice President, Columbus Regional
Healthcare System, Inc.

Comprehensive Community Health Models of Michigan
18 West Michigan Avenue, 3rd Floor
Battle Creek, MI 49017-3604
ph: (616) 963-3736
fx: (616) 962-7747
Contact: Pamela Paul-Shaheen
Director, Operations

Creating a Healthier Macomb
15855 19 Mile Road
Clinton Township, MI 48038
ph: (810) 263-2722
fx: (810) 263-2614
Contact: Kurt Kazanowski
VP, Community Healthcare System
Development

DeKalb County Board of Health
Community Health Promotion Division
P.O. Box 987
Decatur, GA 30031
ph: (404) 508-7845
fx: (404) 294-3842
Contact: Micky Roberts
Health Education Manager

Departmento de Formento a la Salud
Servicios Coordinados De Salud Publica
5 Poniente 1322 Zona Esmerelda
C.P. , MEXICO 72000
ph: 011-52-22-32-80-40
fx: 011-52-22-32-09-38
Contact: Ivette Rivera Guzman
Secretaria de Salud

Departmento de Formento a la Salud
Numero De Oficio 5013/15 Sur No 302
Xochitlan, Puebla, MEXICO 72000
ph: 011-52-22-32-80-40
fx: 011-52-22-32-09-38
Contact: Dr. Eduardo Vazquez Valdes
Subjefatura De Servs. De Salud

Desert Hospital, Palm Springs in Action
P.O. Box 2739
1150 North Indian Canyon Drive
Palm Springs, CA 92262
ph: (619) 323-6305
fx: (619) 323-6825
Contact: Kelley Green
Community Network Coordinator

Developing Principles and Conducting a Community Assessment
6700 North Highway 101
Eureka, CA 95503
ph: (707) 443-9332
fx: (707) 443-8142
Contact: Catherine Krause
Area Vice President for
Home/Community Health

Dominican Network and Health Improvement Partnership
5633 North Lidgerwood
Spokane, WA 99207
ph: (509) 482-2458
fx: (509) 456-6569
Contact: Barbara Savage
VP, Mission/Coordinator Health
Improvement

First Transition
125 North Executive Drive, Suite 355
Brookfield, WI 53005
ph: (414) 821-7107
fx: (414) 821-1492
Contact: Francis Wiesner
Partner

Garrett Countians for a Healthier Year 2000
253 North Fourth Street
Oakland, MD 21550
ph: (301) 334-8122
fx: (301) 334-1014
Contact: Ann Sherrard, RD, MPH
Director of Community Health

Greater Southeast Healthcare System
1310 Southern Avenue
Washington, DC 20032-4692
ph: (202) 574-6076
fx: (612) 232-4864
Contact: Jacquelyn Lendsey
VP, Corp/Community Development

Growing Into Life Task Force
7 Burgundy Road
Aiken, SC 92801
ph: (803) 648-8520
fx: (803) 642-7646
Contact: Karen Papouchado
Coordinator
Contact: Barbara Strack
Coordinator

Health Improvement Partnership
5633 North Lidgerwood
Spokane, WA 99207
ph: (509) 482-2557
fx: (509) 482-2456 or (509) 456-6569
Contact: Dan Baumgarten
President

Health Quest
407 East 3rd Street
Duluth, MN 55805
ph: (218) 726-4486
fx: (218) 726-4383
Contact: Jim Cherveny
Executive Vice President

Healthcare 1999
Healthcare 1999, Old Main Building
Pembroke, NC 28372-1510
ph: (910) 521-6182
Contact: Paul Robertus
Executive Director

HealthEast
MetroEast Program for Health
1690 University Avenue, Suite 220
St. Paul, MN 55104
ph: (612) 232-4819
fx: (612) 232-4834
Contact: Debra Trautman
Senior Director

Healthy Boston
43 Hawkins, Room 3B
Boston, MA 02114
ph: (617) 635-2770
fx: (617) 635-3353
Contact: Jerry Mogul
Operations Manager

Healthy Chico Kids 2000\ Pacific Wellness Institute
California State University, Chico
Building U
Chico, CA 95929-0470
ph: (916) 898-4791
fx: (916) 898-4780
Contact: Linda Zorn
Director

Healthy City Toronto
20 Dundas West, Suite 1036
Toronto, Ontario, CANADA M5G 2C2
ph: (416) 392-0099
fx: (416) 392-0089
Contact: Marilou McPhedran
Consultant

Healthy Communities Initiative of Greater Orlando
458 Virginia Drive
Orlando, FL 32789
ph: (407) 649-6891
fx: (407) 872-8533
Contact: Marilyn King, Chairperson

Healthy Community 2000 of Mesa County
c/o The Civic Forum
P.O. Box 2731
Grand Junction, CO 81501
ph: (970) 241-1064
fx: (970) 241-1912
Contact: Alowetta Terrien
Executive Director

Healthy Mountain Communities
P.O. Box 451
Basalt, CO 81621
ph: (970) 963-5502
fx: (970) 963-5502
Contact: Colin Laird
Coordinator

Healthy Sheboygan County 2000
P.O. Box 442
Sheboygan, WI 53082-0442
ph: (414) 457-1587
fx: (414) 457-1595
Contact: Rae Stager
Vice President of Business and
Market Development

Healthy Valley 2000
Griffin Health Services Corporation
130 Division Street
Derby, CT 06418
ph: (203) 732-7515
fx: (203) 732-7448
Contact: William Powanda
Vice President, Support Services

Kaiser Permanente
975 Sereno Drive
Vallejo, CA 94589
ph: (707) 648-6000
fx: (707) 648-6459
Contact: Steve Graham
Director, Community Health Partnerships

Kanawha Coalition for Community Health Improvement
c/o Charleston Area Medical Center
501 Morris Street
Charleston, WV 25326
ph: (304) 348-7885
fx: (304) 348-6314
Contact: Brenda Sue Grant
Corporate Director, Occupational Health

Kent County Health Department
700 Fuller Avenue., N.E.
Grand Rapids, MI 49503
ph: (616) 336-3020
fx: (616) 336-3884
Contact: Lonnie Barnett
Community Health Planner

Lancaster Fairfield Health Clinic
117 West Wheeling Street
Lancaster, OH 43130
ph: (614) 687-6679
fx: (614) 687-6625
Contact: Ed Sachs
MSA Administrator

Memorial Hospital of South Bend
615 North Michigan Street
South Bend, IN 46601-9986
ph: (219) 282-8604
fx: (219) 282-8606
Contact: Carl Ellison
Vice President

Mercy Hospital
5555 Conner
Detroit, MI 48213
ph: (313) 579-4210
fx: (313) 579-4064
Contact: Brenita Crawford
President/CEO

Mercy Mobile Health Care
60 11th Street
Atlanta, GA 30309
ph: (404) 249-8102
fx: (404) 249-8941
Contact: Mary Hood
Clinic Director

Nashville Healthcare Partnership
Nashville Chamber of Commerce
161 4th Avenue North
Nashville, TN 37219
ph: (615) 259-4728
fx: (615) 256-3074
Contact: Joanne Pulles
Executive Director

Office of Community Partnerships
3555 Olentangy River Road
U.S. Health Corporation
Columbus, OH 43214
ph: (614) 566-5894
fx: (614) 477-8244
Contact: Patsy Methany
Director of Community Health Improvement

Operation Healthy Communities
3247 East 7th Street
Durango, CO 81301
ph: (970) 247-5270
fx: (970) 385-4170
Contact: Lynn Shine
Health Index Coordinator

Orlando Regional Healthcare System
1414 Kuhl Avenue
Orlando, FL 32806-2093
ph: (407) 841-5111, ext. 5059
fx: (407) 872-8533
Contact: Sharon McLearn
Admin. Director, Corporate Communications

Overlook Hospital
99 Beauvior Ave.
Summit, NJ 07901-3595
ph: (908) 522-2836
fx: (908) 522-2324
Contact: Connie Williams
Director, Health Promotion

Paradise Valley Hospital

2400 East 4th Street
National City, CA 91950-2099
ph: (619) 470-4110
fx: (619) 470-4124
Contact: Kathryn Wilson
VP, Community and Outpatient Services
Karen McCabe, Director, Community
Health Services

PRO Hampton County

500 Jackson Avenue
Hampton, SC 29924
ph: (803) 941-1235
fx: (803) 943-3943
Contact: Peggy Parker
Director

San Diego Safe Kids Coalition

Children's Hospital and Health Center
MC 5005
3020 Children's Way
San Diego, CA 92123
ph: (619) 495-7748
fx: (619) 467-1882
Contact: Cheri Fidler
Director, Community Relations

San Luis Valley Community Connections

204 Carson Avenue
Alamosa, CO 81101
ph: (719) 589-9691
fx: (719) 589-5722
Contact: Kandiss Bartlett
Director of Health Communications

Silicon Valley Joint Venture

1922 The Alameda, Suite 217
San Jose, CA 95126
ph: (408) 271-7213
fx: (408) 271-7214
Contact: Laurel Hayler
Executive Director

St. Joseph's Mercy Hospital and Health Services

16931 Nineteen Mile Road
Clinton Township, MI 48038
ph: (810) 263-2880
fx: (810) 263-2859
Contact: Scott Adler
Director, Healthier Image Services

St. Joseph's Mercy Care Services

Metropolitan Atlanta Infectious Disease
Program
60 11th Street
Atlanta, GA 30309
ph: (404) 249-8143
fx: (404) 249-8941
Contact: Nancy Paris
Director

Township of Union Network, Inc.

Union Hospital Corporate Building
695 Chestnut Street
Union, NJ 07083-9302
ph: (908) 687-1900 ext. 2025
fx: (908) 851-2327
Contact: Jim Masterson
President of Community Development

Trend Benders

c/o St. Mary's Hospital
P.O. Box 1628
Grand Junction, CO 81502-1628
ph: (970) 244-1975
fx: (970) 244-2092
Contact: Carolyn Bruce
Director of Planning

Union Township Community Initiative

1000 Galloping Hills Road
Union, NJ 07083
ph: (908) 687-1900 ext. 2025
fx: (908) 851-2327
Contact: Reverend Jim Roberts

Upper Valley Medical Centers

3130 North Dixie Highway
Troy, OH 45356
ph: (513) 332-7441
fx: (513) 339-4055
Contact: Lucy Fess
Director of Community Affairs

Westside Health Authority

5437 West Division
Chicago, IL 60651
ph: (312) 378-0233
fx: (312) 378-5035
Contact: Jacqueline Reed
Executive Director

Advisory Panel Members

We extend our gratitude for the contributions and generosity of the following individuals, all of whom played a major role in this workbook's development.

Gruffie Clough, Consultant
Denver, CO

Ross Conner, Associate Professor
of Urban and Regional Planning
Department of Urban and Regional
Planning
School of Social Ecology
University of California, Irvine
Irvine, CA

Carol D'Onofrio, Professor Emeritus
School of Public Health
University of California, Berkeley
Berkeley, CA

Carl Ellison, Vice President
Office of Community Affairs
Memorial Hospital/Health System
South Bend, IN

Christopher Gates, President
National Civic League
Denver, CO

Karen Glanz, Professor
University of Hawai'i at Manoa
Cancer Research Center of Hawai'i
Honolulu, HI

Steve Graham, Director
Community Health Partnerships
Kaiser Permanente
Vallejo, CA

Trevor Hancock, Public Health
Consultant
Kleinburg, Ontario, Canada

Arthur Himmelman, President
The HIMMELMAN Consulting Group
Minneapolis, MN

Leland Kaiser, President
Kaiser and Associates
Brighton, CO

Marilyn King, Chairperson
Healthy Community Initiative
of Greater Orlando
Winter Park, FL

Jacquelyn Lendsey, Vice President
Corporate and Community Development
Greater Southeast Healthcare System
Washington, DC

Marilou McPhedran, Advocate
Health, Systems and Advocacy
Toronto, Ontario, Canada

Gary Nelson, PhD, Senior Program
Officer
The California Wellness Foundation
Woodland Hills, CA

Tyler Norris, President
Tyler Norris and Associates
Boulder, CO

Amalie Ramirez, DrPH,
Associate Professor
Department of Family Practice
University of Texas
Health Science Center at San Antonio
San Antonio, TX

Sarah Samuels, DrPH, Consultant
Health Programs and Policy
Oakland, CA

Julia Weaver, Director
Healthy Community Programs
National Civic League
Denver, CO

Preface

In the spirit of collaboration, **The California Wellness Foundation** and **The Healthcare Forum** have partnered to develop *Collaborating to Improve Community Health: Workbook and Guide to Best Practices in Creating Healthier Communities and Populations*, designed to support community-based partnerships worldwide in their collaborative efforts.

Throughout this book, jazz is used as a metaphor for community collaboration. The unique art of jazz is a process much like that needed to arrive at a successful community collaboration: individual musicians contribute their distinctive talents and creative flair, which result in a delightful melody that each alone could not create. In this workbook we hope to illustrate how, through the "art" of community collaboration, we can fortify our individual efforts and collectively create more harmonious places to live.

This workbook embodies the experiences, lessons and accomplishments of more than 50 community partnerships across North America as they endeavor to make their neighborhoods healthy places to live, raise families, work and grow. Readers will explore the Core Processes or principal phases involved in mounting a collaborative effort and will become familiar with the essential steps and key players. Using Action Worksheets in the back of each Core Process chapter, your local community effort may benefit from systems fine-tuned by others worldwide. Real-life vignettes sown throughout the workbook will heighten your awareness of successful methods and strategies as they detail the "how-to's" of initiating, maintaining and evaluating community efforts in rural and urban communities throughout United States and beyond.

We would like to take this opportunity to thank the more than 50 leading-edge community partnerships across the country, with additional representatives from Canada and Mexico, who have contributed their time and expertise in the creation of this workbook. In the interest of allowing similar efforts to prosper from their countless lessons and vast community experience, representatives from contributing partnerships submitted information on their collaboration's "Best Practices" in the form of survey responses. (See Appendix A for the survey questions.)

Research Methodology—Identification of Best Practices

Because we lack formal baseline performance data with which to compare best practices in collaboration, the formulation of the best practices within this resource is accumulated advice and wisdom from experts in the field. This workbook does not attempt to create baseline performance data where none exist. Instead we have used expert opinion to generate Core Processes, Critical Success Factors and best practices in community collaboration. Considering that there are less than ample formal benchmarks from which to learn about community collaboration, this workbook is the best expert advice to those who are engaging in and learning from this process daily.

We surveyed efforts across North America that used results-oriented processes involving multisectoral groups working together and sharing resources to improve community health and well-being. The collaborative efforts were also to be focused on programs, policies and strategies that extend beyond medical care and addressed root causes and determinants of good health, such as integrated systems of services, strong local economies and educational opportunities for all.

The Best Practices survey was distributed to 370 community partnerships around North America. In addition to responding to the survey, many of the partnerships were also represented at the Best Practices Process Design Meeting that took place at The Healthcare Forum's 1996 Healthier Communities Summit. At this collaborative full-day design session, experts representing 45 communities discussed successful strategies and techniques in collaboration. Participants in this meeting shared their community's ideas with representatives of other partnerships while exchanging "trade secrets" from their collective experience, which they could apply to their own efforts. The rich array of lessons and experience gleaned from this summit of community leaders has been compiled in this workbook.

Metaphor

Many aspects of collaboration allow for comparison with jazz . Improvisation is perhaps the most obvious. Once a jazz musician becomes familiar with the basis of this colorful art form—rhythm, harmony and structure—he may explore countless variations of "the norm." Similarly, stakeholders in a community collaboration need to understand the structure their effort will be based on. From that juncture they are free to "improvise" or engage in a unique arrangement of tasks to improve their community.

Improvisation, however random it may seem to the observer, is best done within a group of people who understand one another. The best jazz groups share clear communication through verbal or physical signs to lead them through the stirring improvisational stages of their arrangements. Musicians support each other through solos, knowing that they too will be supported when the time is right. Jazz is a truly collective creation, with musicians showcasing each other's talents, adding strength and support wherever necessary. Community members also feed off each other's creativity within a collaborative process. Many of the best ideas in both the musical and collaborative realms conform strictly to the overall structure and principles of their respective schools and yet use the unique blend of intermingling ingredients to their advantage. Talents of one group member complement those of another, reinforcing each member's strengths to make the group a more powerful working unit.

The essence of improvisation also makes for unique results. Just as two jazz groups improvising will never sound alike, distinct communities working toward common goals will always yield different results. We must learn to be aware of the skills and abilities of each of our members so that we can put forth the strongest blend of talents the group has to offer. Veteran Minneapolis jazz bassist Biddy Bastien asserts that a group can play at a level only slightly above the competence of its least knowledgeable member. Improvisation, therefore, also involves being responsive to local circumstances and seeing them as ingredients to carefully combine for a successful collaboration.

If we look at organizing the effort—the basis for the structure we have developed in this workbook—as the sheet music to our "community jazz," the remaining Core Processes become the rhythms and harmonies essential to jazz: vital to the sound but subject to each musician's creative whims. As you read, keep in mind that we are giving you the sheet music and theory in this workbook but that it will be up to you and your community to breathe life into that knowledge and create your own unique sound.

> Improvisation, therefore, also involves being responsive to local circumstances and seeing them as ingredients to carefully combine for a successful collaboration.

Acknowledgments

We are grateful to The California Wellness Foundation for providing full funding for the development of this workbook and especially to Gary Nelson, PhD, for making it happen. The foundation has a long history of commitment and of contributing to the building of healthy communities throughout California. The California Wellness Foundation's Health Improvement Initiative, which funded this workbook, is a new five-year, $20,000,000 effort to enhance population health through comprehensive integrated systems of community-based preventive services.

A special thanks to Micky Roberts and Barbara Strack, our "community editors," and all of the individuals who took time out of their busy schedules to be interviewed for the four case studies in this workbook. We also would like to acknowledge our ongoing appreciation of members of the National Civic League and Tyler Norris of Tyler Norris and Associates, along with countless others who have worked closely with The Healthcare Forum to promote and advance the philosophy of Healthier Communities over the years.

This workbook is intended to serve as a practical tool for the many communities working collaboratively for a better future throughout the state of California and around the world.

June 1997
San Francisco, California

Kathryn E. Johnson
Wynne Grossman
Anne Cassidy

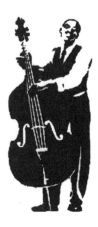

The Editors

Kathryn E. Johnson

Kathryn Johnson is president and chief executive officer of The Healthcare Forum, a national and international not-for-profit healthcare association based in San Francisco, California. The Forum provides healthcare leaders and managers with high-quality educational and informational products and services. The vision of the organization is to create healthier communities by engaging leaders in building new visions and models of care.

The Healthcare Forum fulfills its vision by publishing *The Healthcare Forum Journal*, presenting executive education conferences, and sponsoring a major annual meeting with educational programming. The Healthcare Forum Foundation Leadership Center conducts applied research, and recognizes and honors excellence in the healthcare field through various awards and programs.

Johnson graduated from Indiana University and earned her master's degree in organizational behavior at Boston University. Johnson served as the director of management development at Massachusetts General Hospital in Boston from 1969 to 1976. In 1976 she joined the Association of Western Hospitals, which reorganized and became The Healthcare Forum in 1987.

In 1984, Johnson was awarded a three-year Kellogg National Leadership Fellowship. In 1992, she was selected Woman of the Year by the Women Health Care Executives of Northern California. In 1993, she received the Key Award, the highest honor bestowed by the American Society of Association Executives.

Wynne Grossman

Wynne Grossman is director of research and development for The Healthcare Forum and is responsible for the development of The Forum's Applied Research Agenda. Research projects include the following: Bridging the Leadership Gap; Transforming Healthcare Delivery: Building Learning Organizations by Linking Systems Thinking and Total Quality; What Creates Health? Individuals and

Communities Respond; Best Practices for Community Health Partnerships; and the Accelerating Community Transformation project.

Products include The Forum's three Learning Labs—Mastering the Transition to Capitation; Risky Business: Mastering the New Business of Health; the Community Builder: Strategies for Improving Quality of Life; The Learning Advantage: A Tool for Building Learning Organizations; The Healthier Communities Action Kit; The Healthier Community Award; The Sustaining Community-Based Initiatives Workbooks; and the forthcoming Outcomes Toolkit. Conferences include Transforming Healthcare Delivery and Breakthrough Performance.

Grossman has a master's degree in community organization, planning and administration from the University of California at Berkeley. She was formerly the vice president of Saybrook Institute in San Francisco, the director of marketing for Gladman Hospital in Oakland, and the director of development and alumni relations for the Haas School of Business at the University of California at Berkeley.

Anne Cassidy

Anne Cassidy is the Healthier Communities Manager for The Healthcare Forum. She works with all Healthier Communities initiatives at The Forum.

Cassidy also coordinated the Sustaining Community-Based Initiatives project funded by the Kellogg Foundation, which produced four learning modules designed to build capacity within community-based organizations. The goal of the project was to enable community leaders to sustain their efforts at improving health and well-being in their communities.

Currently, Cassidy is the project manager for the Accelerating Community Transformation project and for the development of the Outcomes Toolkit, designed to assist communities in monitoring the results of their collaborative efforts to improve overall health and quality of life.

Cassidy earned a B.A. in Spanish from Dickinson College in Carlisle, Pennsylvania. She joined The Healthcare Forum after working for Charles Schwab & Co., Inc., where she managed relations between sales and compliance within Schwab Institutional. She also spent two years as a Peace Corps volunteer in Central America, where she worked promoting adult literacy and basic nutritional awareness throughout western Honduras.

The Core Processes in Community Collaboration

Convening the Community

- Include diverse stakeholders
- Acknowledge the "spark" or catalyst of the process
- Frame both the process and desired outcomes to generate buy-in from all stakeholders
- Ensure credibility by including visible as well as "non-traditional" leaders

Creating a Shared Vision

- Develop the shared vision via consensus
- Distinguish the shared vision from shared values
- Invite all stakeholders to continually re-create and refine their shared vision
- Encourage stakeholders to think big!

Monitoring and Adjusting

- Mutually agree on benchmarks and outcomes
- Build in monitoring mechanisms from the outset
- Use multiple methods to gather data
- Enable stakeholders themselves to monitor progress and identify roadblocks
- Continuously document, share and celebrate progress developments
- Use findings to immediately improve the effort

Organizing the Effort

- Clarify and facilitate resource commitments (time, money) by all stakeholders
- Acknowledge unique contributions by all stakeholders
- Agree on processes, procedures and roles
- Develop facilitative leadership capacity for all phases in the process

Assessing Current Realities and Trends

- Measure assets, not just needs or liabilities
- Identify resources that will ensure assessment is effective
- Link assessment to vision, action and outcomes
- Gather relevant and useful information, not just easy-to-find data
- Frame questions from multiple points of view

Doing the Job

- Link "doing" with vision, assessment, action planning and outcomes
- Time and link actions so they are synergistic and systemic
- Balance attention to both short- and long-term actions
- Anticipate and address obstacles
- Capitalize on financial incentives such as pooled funding

Action Planning

- Ensure that actions are strategic and leverage-based
- Facilitate ownership by clarifying realistic roles and responsibilities
- Include ambitious and longer-term actions as well as short-term, "small wins"
- Define actions in terms of specific and detailed tasks, tactics and objectives
- Anticipate and plan for training and resources

Introduction

How to Use This Workbook

Community collaboration, like jazz, is both a science and an art. As scientists, we build upon a base of knowledge developed by others. As artists, we must rely on our own creativity to address the needs of our communities, scrutinizing our unique situation and crafting appropriate solutions. This requires a flair for organizing and an intimacy with the community to understand what we need to better serve ourselves and our neighbors.

This workbook is not intended to serve as a "how-to guide." Instead it is intended to provide leaders of collaborative efforts with a framework for guiding your work to improve community health and well-being.

The seven Core Processes that compose this framework are essential to every community collaboration. Our research shows that all successful collaborations engage in all of these seven processes, whether the collaborations are formed to address crime in the community or inadequate prenatal care of a particular population. However, not all successful efforts engage in the processes in the order in which they appear in this workbook. In fact, the most successful collaborations move in, out and among the Core Processes, depending on what feels right at the time. It is not necessary to start by organizing the effort or convening the community. Collaborations often start with an assessment process or with a group of individuals doing something in response to a problem.

Many successful collaborations engage in multiple Core Processes simultaneously. The timing and sequence of what you do depends on the needs and circumstances within your particular community. The way your partnership moves through the Core Processes will determine your community's jazz.

This workbook will give you an outline of each Core Process and describe, in detail, steps that will help you lead your community to successful outcomes.

> Wherever you are in your effort, realize now that a community whose citizens act collaboratively in realizing a shared vision is on the road to reaping great rewards.

Whether you have talked about community problems with friends over dinner or have already engaged in full-fledged community collaboration, the *Collaborating to Improve Community Health: Workbook and Guide* will give you useful information. Regardless of the stage your community is in, you have recognized that a healthy community is worth striving for and, by picking up this workbook, are interested in learning from the experiences—good and bad—of fellow community leaders. Wherever you are in your effort, realize now that a community whose citizens act collaboratively in realizing a shared vision is on the road to reaping great rewards.

Please consider this workbook to be a menu—*not* a blueprint. You must decide how your collaboration engages in each Core Process. Leonard Duhl, MD, one of the key initiators of the World Health Organization's "Healthy Cities" program, advises:

> The various participants (must) define the program. All I say is that you have to start someplace. You have to begin to look at it in an ecological and systemic way. You have to involve people. You have to start thinking of values of equity and participation. Beyond that, you can start wherever you want.

Your starting point is up to you. But remember that it will be difficult to sustain your effort unless your group has an organizing structure, the right people participating, a shared vision, a means of assessing the current situation, an appropriate plan of action, a way to do the work and to monitor your results.

You can use this book to

- Learn the "how-to's" within each Core Process of community collaboration by following the steps in each clearly detailed diagram

- Assist you in the process through the use of the Action Worksheets as tools

- Gain insight into "how" to engage in each practice through real-life vignettes from other community leaders across the country

- Jump-start a lagging community collaboration with new strategies and initiatives

- Pick and choose detailed Core Processes that are appropriate for your particular stage in collaboration (if you have successfully convened your community, move on to the chapter on creating a shared vision)

- Get clarification on a particular part of the collaborative process

- Gather additional resources on community assessment, collaboration and coalition building and the Healthy Communities movement by using the resource sections in the back of the workbook

- Make new contacts and share information with the other collaborative efforts around the country

- Spread the word about collaboration in your community and beyond, using the overheads provided in this workbook

Rather than taking a fragmented, one-on-one approach to community problems, communities across America have begun to collaborate.

A Word or Two About Collaboration

As a society we have become extremely individualistic in the last few decades. The 1980s were accompanied by a "me first" attitude, but trends show the pendulum beginning to swing back in the other direction. Rather than taking a fragmented, one-on-one approach to community problems, communities across America have begun to collaborate.

Many different models of collaboration are emerging. These include strategic alliances and partnerships of two to three stakeholders (sectors of the community: public, private, religious, etc.), coalitions of 10 or more stakeholders, and community-wide efforts that engage numerous organizations (from non-profit to the corporate sector) as well as the public. These initiatives may have one objective, such as addressing neighborhood vandalism, or they may be working together to address a variety of issues and objectives.

Regardless of the number of stakeholders and the number of objectives, these collaborative efforts are based on a common set of "success factors." These basic principles appear throughout this workbook. Successful collaborative efforts

- Are open, inclusive and diverse

- Identify and build upon individual, organizational and community assets and strengths

- Empower stakeholders in a positive, non-threatening way

- Are based on a compelling, shared vision

- Are based on strategies and tactics that directly relate to the vision.

- Are well timed

- Are based on tangible, visible commitments of resources by the stakeholders
- Have the power to implement their own recommendations
- Use consensus to reach desired outcomes
- Value the "process" as well as the "results"
- Measure outcomes regularly
- Define goals and objectives
- Celebrate milestones and achievements
- Sustain the momentum
- Require patience

Among the myriad strategies, the collaborative process should embody two essential concepts: systems thinking and sustainability. Peter Senge, director of the Center for Organizational Learning at MIT's Sloan School of Management, says, "Today's problems come from yesterday's solutions." Many short-sighted collaborations have yielded disastrous results. To plan for the future it is essential that our vision take a systems approach and consider the "big picture." We need to incorporate a systemic view of societal challenges that sees our effort as part of a larger interrelated system, rather than as a fragmented process.

According to Art Kleiner, co-author with Senge and others of *The Fifth Discipline Fieldbook*:

> A system is a perceived whole whose elements "hang together" because they continually affect each other over time and operate toward a common purpose. The word descends from the Greek verb *sunistanai*, which originally meant "to cause to stand together." As this origin suggests, the structure of a system includes the quality of perception with which you, the observer, cause it to stand together.

> Examples of systems include biological organisms (including human bodies), the atmosphere, diseases, ecological niches, factories, chemical reactions, political entities, communities, industries, families, teams—and all organizations. You and your work are probably elements of dozens of different systems.

(Copyright ©1990, Bantam Doubleday Dell. Reprinted with permission.)

Sustainability is also critical to the success of all community collaborations. Many efforts begin partnerships and programs without benefit of structural, operational and relational mechanisms to build the capacity necessary to support the effort over time. Rather than being viewed simply as projects to complete in the short term, community collaborative efforts should be viewed as long-term efforts whose core human, social and economic resources should be actively nurtured and continuously renewed as a community asset. Without a long-term, sustaining focus, these efforts may not realize their vision or achieve their intended objectives.

Rather than being viewed simply as projects to complete in the short-term, community collaborative efforts should be viewed as long-term efforts whose core human, social and economic resources should be actively nurtured and continuously renewed as a community asset.

Workbook Structure

This workbook is organized around seven Core Processes (a series of interrelated activities or events that convert inputs into results—successful collaboration outcomes). One of these Core Processes, organizing the effort, acts as a "Metaprocess" (foundation or structure that fortifies the remaining six Core Processes). Each Core Process chapter has a diagram that leads you through a visual representation of the essential steps and key players involved. After a brief overview, each chapter delves into a Core Process, providing real-life vignettes of "Best Practices." Action Worksheets allow you to use local community information to engage actively in what you have read and apply the knowledge to your own local effort. Potential Pitfalls in each of the Core Processes serve as thought-provokers. Case studies lead you through steps taken by communities as they wend their way through Core Processes toward successful outcomes. Two communities are rural, two are urban. A broad geographic representation gives examples that all readers can relate to. The final section in the workbook includes appendixes, a glossary, a bibliography organized by workbook section and a variety of other resources related to our topic.

Core Process Diagram Overview

Critical Success Factors in each Core Process appear at the top of each diagram. All Critical Success Factors are actions and conditions that are essential for Core Process development. You may find your partnership will establish more Critical Success Factors for each Core Process than appear in this workbook.

Each diagram illustrates the degree of process involvement by the following groups:

- Coordinator and Staff: Individuals, often hired by the partnership, who take care of many administrative and organizational concerns of the effort. The staff must have good group and organizational process skills and a community development philosophy.

- Coordinating Committee: A group of 10 to 15 people who are willing to lead the effort and invest substantial time in at least the developmental phase of the initiative. It is essential that this group be representative of the diversity of the entire community and should have at least one member from each major community sector.

- Stakeholders: People who join your effort from all ranks of the community. Stakeholders can be concerned individuals or established community groups. On each diagram we represent all community stakeholders by four generic groups (One, Two, Three and Four) that stand for organizational as well as individual partners. In all likelihood, your effort may have more than four stakeholder groups.

Each step within a Core Process is spearheaded by one of the groups in the partnership. In the Core Process diagrams, each step appears in the column of the initiator of that step. Musical notes on the same horizontal axis represent the collaboration of other partners in the step.

You will note that steps detailed within each Core Process follow a particular sequence (whereas Core Processes themselves need not be in a particular order) and sometimes accompany important "decision points," completion of which ensures readiness to move on to the next step. Following the steps in the sequence they appear will enhance your chances for success. For example, under the Core Process organizing the effort, an agreed-upon mission and set of principles provide a solid foundation for future work. If you do not take the time to build this foundation early on, your initiative may find itself on shaky ground later.

Core Processes Overview

Organizing the Effort

Organizing the effort acts as the Metaprocess, or sheet music, that lies at the heart of the other Core Processes. In organizing the effort, the Coordinating Committee and staff create the mechanisms, agreements, policies and procedures that support the entire partnership and "operationalize" multisectoral collaboration. Further, they link the Core Processes together so they are synergistic and complementary.

Convening the Community

This Core Process describes steps necessary for organizing and mobilizing the community in a collaborative effort to improve community health and quality of life. It details the importance of including a wide array of community sectors to ensure representation of diverse viewpoints.

Creating a Shared Vision

In this Core Process, stakeholders, staff and Coordinating Committee develop a bold, vivid picture of what they would like their community's quality of life to be. The steps within the chapter specify how to arrive at your community's compelling shared vision.

Assessing Current Realities and Trends

This Core Process includes steps necessary for gathering accurate, meaningful information about key dimensions and determinants of health. Assessment should be tailored to the purpose and desired outcomes of the partnership, and create opportunities for insight as well as action by stakeholders, the Committee and the public. It is also a basis for measuring the effect (direct and indirect) of the effort on population health.

Action Planning

In this Core Process, the Coordinating Committee—with input from stakeholders and staff—develops and documents a coherent, user-friendly action plan. The plan describes the partnership's goals for improving health, its objectives, and high-leverage strategies and methods it will use to address these goals and objectives. It may contain programs, initiatives and projects. The plan assigns Committee members, staff and stakeholders to each goal or program, and defines the time frame for action. Most important, the plan describes how programs and projects will be linked so that they are synergistic.

Doing the Job

This is the implementation phase of the effort. The partnership must be "strategic" in how it carries out initiatives and projects specified in the action plan. Because conditions change—often dramatically—after the action plan is developed, projects are timed, linked, coordinated and ultimately rolled out so they capitalize on political, economic and social resources and other opportunities. These steps are circular, and they overlap synergistically.

Monitoring and Adjusting

In this Core Process, all stakeholders play a role in measuring both the process and outcomes of the partnership. Information is gathered using a variety of tools and formats, formally and informally. Most important, the information gathered is used by stakeholders and the Committee to improve the partnership.

Case Studies and Resource
Section Overview

Case Studies

This section includes in-depth case studies of the following four collaborative efforts across the country:

Growing Into Life, Aiken, South Carolina
Bethel New Life, Chicago, Illinois
Healthy Community 2000 of Mesa County, Grand Junction, Colorado
Healthy Communities Initiative of Greater Orlando, Orlando, Florida

Each case study gauges the progress made by partnerships in their journey through Core Processes to act collaboratively in improving the health of their communities. You will note successful strategies that worked well for each effort, in addition to learning from mistakes.

Resources

In addition to the Appendixes and the Glossary (with terms that may be unfamiliar to you), there is a Resources section at the end of the workbook. This section has valuable information for partnerships seeking guidance on collaboration toward Healthier Communities. The Resources include the following:

- Bibliography by Workbook Section

- Additional Resources, further divided in sections on community assessment, collaboration and coalition building, and healthy communities

- Annotated Resources, divided into the same categories

A Final Note

Our goal in providing this workbook is to make it a "user-friendly" resource that anyone, whether a motivated community member or a representative from a well-established partnership, can pick up and find useful. You are not alone in your admirable efforts. Collaboration is going on across the globe in a multitude of ways. Many individuals who we believe excel in their collaborative initiatives toward improved wellness have shared their expertise in this volume. We hope it helps you streamline and capitalize on your efforts, and avoid reinventing the wheel. Good luck in creating your community's jazz.

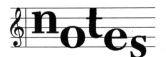

Organizing the Effort

Agree on mission, values and principles

Agree on a process for working together

Design organizational structure

Determine meeting guidelines

Define roles and responsibilities

Create an effective process for communication

Coordinate budget and fund development

Link with other efforts

Celebrate!

Promote the effort

Build the leadership capacity of all stakeholders

Enlist technical assistance and support

Organizing the Effort

Critical Success Factors

- Clarify and facilitate resource commitments (time, money) by all stakeholders
- Acknowledge unique contributions by all stakeholders
- Agree on processes, procedures and roles
- Develop facilitative capacity for all phases in the process

Coordinator and Staff	Coordinating Committee	Stakeholder One	Stakeholder Two	Stakeholder Three	Stakeholder Four
♫	**Step 1** — Agree on mission, values and principles	♫	♫	♫	♫
♫	**Step 2** — Agree on process for working together	♫	♫	♫	♫
	Step 3 — Design organizational structure				
	Step 4 — Determine meeting guidelines				
♫	**Step 5** — Define roles and responsibilities	♫	♫	♫	♫
	Step 6 — Create an effective process for communication				
♫	**Step 7** — Coordinate budget and fund development				
♫	**Step 8** — Link with other efforts				
♫	**Step 9** — Celebrate!				
♫	**Step 10** — Promote the effort	♫	♫	♫	♫
♫	**Step 11** — Build the leadership capacity of all stakeholders				
♫	**Step 12** — Enlist technical assistance and support				

♫ = Step is done by the corresponding partners as well as the initiator

This process was mapped by: Lonnie Barnett, Adele Crocker, Kelley Greene, Micky Roberts, Barbara Savage and Kathryn Wilson

Organizing the Effort

Organizing the effort is the Core Process that lies at the *heart* of the other Core Processes. It acts as a Metaprocess, bridging the gap between each stage of the effort, and serves as the "sheet music" to fortify the creativity of the remaining Core Processes. In organizing the effort, the Committee and staff create mechanisms, agreements, policies and procedures that support the entire partnership and "operationalize" multisectoral collaboration. Further, stakeholders and staff link all processes together so they are synergistic and complementary.

Because working across sectors is distinct from working within one sector or one organization, in organizing the effort the partnership's Coordinating Committee, staff and stakeholders must co-develop mechanisms and processes that are tailor-made and appropriate for this type of "organization." For example, partnerships must build in creative mechanisms for facilitating cross-stakeholder communication, such as frequent meetings. This enables trust and commitment to grow in efforts where participants are volunteering their time and where there may be "turfism."

Partnerships must also build in mechanisms and policies that ensure learning, "upstream" thinking and action, shared leadership, accountability to the public, celebration and renewal.

Finally, partnerships must continually create new policies and mechanisms. As the partnership moves from one phase to the next, new structures and agreements are needed to ensure success. If trust and true commitment to a shared vision of community wellness have been established as fundamental tenets of the collaborative process from the outset, these revisions should prove less challenging.

These procedures and agreements are essential in partnerships because how community leaders work together effectively to address shared concerns is as important as whether the initiative improves population health.

1. Agree on the mission, values and principles of the effort.

The first step in organizing the effort is gaining the agreement of the staff, Coordinating Committee and stakeholders on the effort's mission, values and principles. This step can be time-consuming, but is essential before the effort can move forward. (A substep here, often dictated by reality, is sometimes reaching the agreement within the Coordinating Committee and then ensuring that stakeholders concur.) Steps include the following:

- Identify vehicles for arriving at these agreements (meetings, retreats)

- Validate agreements with all stakeholders

- Document agreements using a variety of formats

- Agree on the value of the process itself (not simply the outcomes)

"We decided to invite the community to treat staff as resource partners as opposed to prescribing experts."

— Micky Roberts

Agreeing on the mission, values and principles of the effort, we decided to invite the community to treat staff as resource partners as opposed to prescribing experts. The vehicle for allowing this kind of interaction to take place included a survey of the community. In each group we included staff, Coordinating Committee members, and stakeholders. Each team followed a specific course, identifying various housing patterns, businesses, schools, recreational facilities, etc. Within each, one person recorded the discussion in an attempt to identify the strengths and challenges that were identified in specific areas. Other meetings followed monthly that built on discussions with groups sharing observations about community strengths and weaknesses. From these meetings the group decided to establish a purpose and to ensure that we would have stakeholders from throughout the community. We then used the community wheel (CSAP "Assessing Breadth, Depth and Scope") exercise to identify different sectors and organization participation critical to the success of the coalition's formulation.

—Micky Roberts, Clarkston Health Collaborative, Clarkston, Georgia

(Image above is taken from "Identifying Training and Technical Assistance Needs in Community Coalitions: A Developmental Approach," by Paul Florin, et al. *Health Education Research*, 8. Reprinted with permission.)

Sample Ground Rules for Collaborative Meetings

Many collaborative efforts find it useful to create ground rules for group behavior and meetings. Agreeing to abide by group rules can help members develop group norms and design an ideal environment where everyone feels comfortable.

You may create one set of ground rules that apply to all meetings, or create special ground rules for different occasions. Make sure all participants have input into creating or approving ground rules; give each person a copy, or post them on large newsprint in a visible location. Here are some sample ground rules that you may use to generate your own ideas

As a group, members of our collaborative effort agree to

1. Share information about our groups and learn from others about theirs.
2. Be respectful of the way that others want us to treat them. We will not demean, devalue, or in any way put down people. No making jokes at the expense of others.
3. Give new voices a chance. Do not dominate the discussion.
4. Combat and correct misinformation about the myths and stereotypes about our own and other groups.
5. Keep our discussions here confidential. Respect people's privacy.
6. Treat our own and other people's ideas and emotions with respect.
7. Listen and don't interrupt while one person speaks.
8. Agree to disagree, but respect everyone's feelings.
9. Treat people as individuals, not as representatives of an entire group.
10. Respect and appreciate each other's uniqueness.

2. Agree on a process for working together.

Based on these agreements, the Coordinating Committee, with stakeholder and staff input, develops an explicit process for collaborating and sharing accountability and leadership. The Committee should do the following:

- Consider engaging a neutral process consultant or facilitator

- Determine how and when training and orientation will be provided

- Develop a mechanism for consensus-based decision-making and ground rules for meetings (see sample ground rules)

- Develop a mechanism for ongoing documentation

- Develop a mechanism for conflict resolution

The use of consultation is an effective way to discuss an issue. Consultation ensures that all participate in the deliberations. Everyone is equal. All opinions, whether agreed with or not, are considered. All must listen courteously to what is being said by the speaker. We concentrate on the issue, not the person speaking. Once an idea, thought or plan is presented, it belongs to the group. The group owns the idea. Therefore, when suggestions or changes are made, it is much easier to do.

— Adele Crocker, Healthy Flin Flon, Canada

"Once an idea, thought or plan is presented, it belongs to the group. The group owns the idea. Therefore, when suggestions or changes are made, it is much easier to do."

—Adele Crocker

3. Design organizational structure.

Every effort needs to develop a structure for dividing up the labor and clarifying lines of authority, a structure that is appropriate for its community, values and desired outcomes. Although this structure varies from effort to effort, it is important to keep it simple. Some typical steps and considerations in developing the structure are as follows:

- Benchmark the organizational structures of exemplary efforts
- Clarify how each "function" relates to other functions
- Enable "functions" to link and collaborate easily
- Determine the number of participants on the Committee
- Determine the number of stakeholders for the overall effort
- Form Action Teams or committees to address key functions
- Designate leaders and co-leaders for each Action Team
- Create a process for continually adding new members as needed

 We decided to remain as "transparent" an organization as possible, except where the public needed to see a cohesive effort. Our goal is to facilitate the organization and implementation of efforts, and then to let the leaders of those ventures take the credit. We find a chairperson every two years. We have leaned toward high-profile elected officials who can weather opposition with a look, and we back them up with strong technical support.

— Karen Papouchado, Growing Into Life, Aiken, South Carolina

Not surprisingly, a finding from studies of coalitions and block associations conducted by David Chavis and others (1987) revealed that the more structured and routinized an effort was, the more likely that effort was to achieve longevity.

4. Determine meeting guidelines.

Meetings are one way that partnerships do the important work of making decisions, building trust among stakeholders and strategizing solutions. Since partnership meetings often include people who have no prior experience working together, and meetings are the mechanism for moving forward, the Committee needs to

- Send letters of invitation before each meeting
- Send minutes or summaries after each meeting
- Use a variety of meeting formats (in person, phone conferences, etc.)
- Establish a standard meeting format that encourages participation
- Hold stakeholder meetings regularly
- Agree on timeline for meetings
- Rotate meetings to include various groups
- Identify community participants to chair or co-facilitate the meetings with paid staff

We hold quarterly meetings that are reminiscent of the 60s in their quality of "happening." Major systems problems get solved through these two-hour exercises in managed chaos. New people are assimilated into the system. Triumphs are celebrated, and people encountering obstacles are reminded of our motto: "Over, under, around, and through." We have not yet found a problem that could not be addressed through one or more of these techniques.

> "'Over, under, around, and through.' We have not yet found a problem that could not be addressed through one or more of these techniques."
>
> — Karen Papouchado

5. Define roles and responsibilities.

The Coordinating Committee, with staff and stakeholder input, also needs to make explicit the roles and responsibilities of all participants. Steps include the following:

- Agree on contributions and expectations of partners
- Define authority of staff, Committee members, and stakeholders

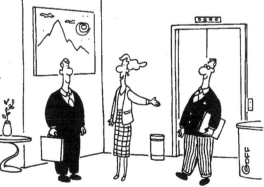

"I'D LIKE YOU TO MEET 20% OF THE REASON FOR OUR TEAM'S SUCCESS."

> *"Stakeholders should be worker bees to engender their ownership and talents."*
>
> — Kelley Green

- Create mechanism to share risks, rewards, responsibilities
- Define role and authority of Action Teams
- Document roles and responsibility agreements
- Install a Coordinating Committee that is representative of the community
- Agree on fiduciary responsibilities

> ☞ *Tip: Follow all of the steps in organizing the effort process, but don't spend too much time at any one of them. The project coordinators should support the project, but should not do all of the footwork. Other stakeholders should be worker bees to engender their ownership and talents.*
>
> — Kelley Green, Palm Springs in Action - California Healthy Cities Project, Palm Springs, California

6. Create an effective process for communication.

This includes communication within the effort and among the effort and the media, public and other interested parties. The process should include the following steps:

- Develop a compelling message
- Identify vehicles for communicating (meetings, newsletters, brochures, PSAs)
- Hold meetings with editorial boards
- Be specific!
- Agree on who should receive communications
- Ensure that communications (quality, frequency) are adequate but not overwhelming

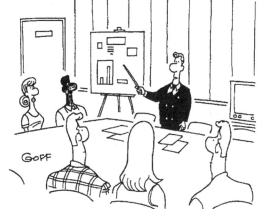

"THIS IS THE GOAL OUR PARTNERSHIP WOULD SORT OF LIKE TO REACH SOMETIME OR OTHER."

Initial planning for Healthy Valley 2000 included development of a Marketing Plan covering at least 6 to 12 months. This included establishment of a Marketing Committee. The role of the Marketing Committee is to set strategic direction. The principal responsibility of the Marketing Committee is to ensure broad community awareness of the effort: its vision, mission, and goals; progress and achievement of initiatives and contribution of the project and initiatives to improving the health and quality of life of the community and its residents. Related responsibilities are to ensure that all communications and events achieve a high standard for quality and to ensure the project and community regularly celebrate successes through planned activities and events. The marketing component has contributed greatly to the success of the project, resulted in additional stakeholders and the support of government leaders, and has been a major factor in acquiring grants and sponsors.

— Bill Powanda, Healthy Valley 2000, Derby, Connecticut

7. Coordinate budget and fund development.

Although people—not money—are arguably the key ingredients for success, most efforts require money to finance the partnership itself as well as the projects or initiatives launched by the collaborative. The Committee should

- Determine which funds are needed for the day-to-day operations of the partnership (including staff, consultants, office space and supplies)

- Determine which funds are needed for projects and initiatives

- Research funding sources (foundations, stakeholders, government agencies, etc.)

- Prepare, submit and track proposals

- Meet with potential funders as needed to secure commitments

- Follow up on commitments

- Monitor partnerships and project budgets to ensure they are on track

- Prepare financial analyses as needed

It is obvious that each initiative's budget will be unique. Many suggestions within this workbook assume the partnership has at least limited funding. Although human resources will be your effort's back-bone and many partnerships scrape by without a great deal of money, you will most likely have certain financial needs. If your initiative is not financially secure, time spent researching funding strategies might be a wise investment.

8. Link with other efforts.

The Committee needs to create a viable process not only for the partnership to do its *own* work but for linking with other collaborative efforts in the community. Considering that it is easy for partnerships to become absorbed in their own desired outcomes, they need to create a formal process for communicating with—and even building off of—other initiatives.

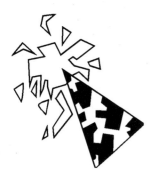

9. Celebrate!

Collaborating is hard work, and the best way to keep it going is to celebrate. Although spontaneous celebrations are wonderful, the Committee needs to make sure that celebration is built into the partnership. Members need to be as detailed about celebrating as they are about actions they want to take together, and

- Clearly identify what you are celebrating
- Create a process for experiencing short-term successes
- Help participants put heart and soul into efforts
- Celebrate launching with a dinner and recognition kick-off
- Celebrate successes (partying, awarding and recognizing)

 Meeting over a long period of time, staff members easily see the success in group development as well as in following and achieving benchmarks for coalition formation and development. However, community coalitions grow weary of meetings and may not perceive benchmarks as actions and/or achievements. In order to address these frustrations, we interject opportunities for "high profile" community-based actions such as health fairs, screenings, recognition banquets, etc. This can happen at any time in the process, based on the collaborative's "mood." This has also included a launching dinner, where those who filled out community matrix forms [see Action Worksheets for convening the community] were invited back. The invitation is open-ended for all participants and members are encouraged to invite others, and if they cannot attend they ask someone to attend in their place.

— Micky Roberts, Clarkston Health Collaborative, Clarkston, Georgia

Another means of celebration is recognition:

 The Westside Health Authority, a community-based organization in Chicago, Illinois, recognizes community members who share resources, gifts and talents with each other in a variety of ways. They often organize neighborhood dinners and other community events and will specially recognize groups and individuals at monthly membership meetings. Local media sources also feature the group's Wellness Initiatives periodically. This recognition not only makes community members feel good about their contributions but also spreads word of their accomplishments nationwide, proven by the fact that they frequently receive inquiries from around the country.

— Jacqueline Reed, Westside Health Authority, Chicago, Illinois

10. Promote the effort.

Members of the public need to be aware of the partnership's accomplishments and challenges. This gives them a chance to comment on or join the process as needed. Stakeholders also benefit from promotion; it enables them to see that they are part of something that is going places, and to identify with the partnership as a whole. In promoting the effort, the Committee and staff should

- Capitalize on stakeholders' relationships with the media

- Coordinate all communications by the initiative with the community

- Coordinate all communication within the initiative

- Conduct ongoing publicity (periodic mailings to VIPs, brochures, press releases, PSAs, etc.)

 We invited members of the media to be stakeholders so they would have a vested interest in promoting the effort. We made follow-up phone calls on the day of the events to back up the media alerts sent out four and two days prior to events. We have had good TV and newspaper coverage. We established personal relationships with reporters, photographers and news anchors. We send copies of newspaper coverage out with our meeting notices and indicate which TV stations covered which events.

— Kelley Green, Palm Springs in Action - California Healthy Cities Project, Palm Springs, California

> "We invited members of the media to be stakeholders so they would have a vested interest in promoting the effort."
> —Kelley Green

"In an effort to enable all Communities Alive! volunteers to feel adequately prepared for the task they have volunteered to undertake, that of creating a healthier community, it was decided that some form of 'basic training' was necessary."

— Lucy Fess

11. Build the leadership capacity of all stakeholders.

Commitment by stakeholders to the goals of the effort is essential for success. But collaboration requires a unique set of skills, skills that stakeholders need to learn and practice. The Committee and staff need to provide these opportunities and consider these steps:

- Define the set of skills and knowledge needed for all stakeholders

- Define the set of skills and knowledge needed for successful participation in Action Teams

- Define the set of skills and knowledge needed for successful leadership (Committee or Team chairs)

- Identify organizations and people who can assist in leadership development

- Agree on format for leadership development (training, presentations, retreats, workbooks, etc.)

- Gain the commitment of all stakeholders to continually building their abilities to lead

- Ensure that there is adequate follow-up training or education

 In an effort to enable all Communities Alive! volunteers to feel adequately prepared for the task they have volunteered to undertake, that of creating a healthier community, it was decided that some form of "basic training" was necessary. . . . The Training Support Team identified eight volunteers who agreed to act as "trainers." Although each of these individuals possess their own area of expertise, it was felt that standardized delivery was necessary when the Community Leadership Training was offered to the community. Topics covered during the "train the trainer" sessions were (1) Team Building, (2) Problem Solving, (3) How to Handle Change, and (4) Facilitation/Conducting an Exchange Meeting.

— Lucy Fess, Upper Valley Medical Center, Troy, Ohio

12. Enlist technical assistance and support.

Every effort encounters roadblocks and critical crossroads. It is important that members be as self-reliant as possible in addressing and overcoming these, but it is also important to know when and how to get much-needed assistance. Too often, "rugged individualism" gets in the way and partnerships don't want to admit they are experiencing problems.

The Committee needs to

- Develop a process for determining if outside help is needed

- Inventory resources (organizations, consultants, publications, conferences, etc.) that can help

- Access those resources

- Determine whether and how the outside experts helped the community in problem-solving

▼

Organizing the effort needs to successfully tie all Core Processes together. The "sheet music" needs to fortify the creativity of the remaining Core Processes. Working together, the Committee, staff and stakeholders must create and implement procedures that support the entire partnership and "operationalize" multisectoral collaboration.

Organizing must flow freely through the Core Processes, contributing to and complementing those processes: convening the community; creating a shared vision; assessing current realities and trends; action planning; doing the job; and monitoring and adjusting. As its structure will govern all future activities and ramifications of the effort, it must be amenable to all stakeholders and will therefore take considerable time and effort to create.

Successfully organizing the effort also means recognizing and capitalizing on the unique contributions of all stakeholders, Committee members and staff. Remember that successful organizing is like improvisation, which involves being responsive to local circumstances and seeing them as ingredients to carefully combine for a successful collaboration.

ACTION WORKSHEET

Potential Pitfalls and Strategies

Use the following worksheet as a way to brainstorm solutions for obstacles that might otherwise undermine your efforts.

Potential Pitfalls	Possible Strategies for Bypassing Pitfalls
1. Lack of resources to hire a neutral facilitator	• Contact agencies in nearby communities for suggestions of skilled facilitators whose services might be contributed. • Seek resources to hire a facilitator from community businesses, or a state or national agency that supports the development of community partnerships. • Agree on process and ground rules to be followed and ask a member of the community to help adhere to these guidelines.
2. Lack of agreement on mission	
3. Competition by stakeholders to run meetings	
4. Difficulty linking with other efforts due to competition or turfism	
5. Celebration of small successes seen as unnecessary	
6. Other Potential Pitfalls . . .	
7.	
8.	

Risk Factors for Collaborative Participation

Take this RISK FACTOR diagnosis to find out which parts of your partnership are "at risk" of discouraging active participation of members and nonmembers and could use a tune-up, and which parts are in good shape. The results may surprise you!

Note: This diagnosis may be of more use to you once your collaborative effort is up and running, but it can provide some interesting insights at any stage of your initiative.

RATE THE FOLLOWING PARTS OF YOUR PARTNERSHIP USING THE SCALE BELOW:

strong/always				weak/never
5	4	3	2	1

1. Clarity of Your Vision and Goals

____ A. Our vision takes into account what is happening in the community.

____ B. The vision and goals are written down.

____ C. Residents and institutions are all aware of the vision and goals of the collaboration.

____ D. We periodically reevaluate and update our vision and goals.

____ E. The activities of the effort are evaluated in relation to our vision and goals.

2. Effectiveness of Your Initiative's Structure

____ A. Our effort has a regular meeting cycle that members can expect.

____ B. There are active committees.

____ C. All members have copies of the by-laws.

_____ D. There is frequent communication among staff, Coordinating Committee and stakeholders.

_____ E. The Coordinating Committee meets regularly with good attendance.

3. Effectiveness of Your Outreach and Communication Tools and Methods

_____ A. The effort has a newsletter or another method of communication that keeps the community regularly updated and informed about its activities.

_____ B. We use a survey or another method to collect information about members' interests, needs and concerns.

_____ C. Survey results are always published and used to guide our projects.

_____ D. The survey is conducted every year or so because the community and residents change.

_____ E. The partnership goes where members are to do outreach, including where people live, shop and work.

4. Effectiveness of Coalition Meetings

_____ A. Stakeholders feel free to speak at meetings without fear of being attacked.

_____ B. The initiative advertises its meetings with sufficient notice by sending out agendas and flyers in advance.

_____ C. Child care and interpreters are provided at meetings when needed.

_____ D. The work of the meeting, as outlined in the agenda, gets accomplished. Meetings start and end on time.

_____ E. Meetings are held in central, convenient and comfortable places and at convenient times for all members.

5. Opportunities for Member Responsibility and Growth

_____ A. The partnership makes a conscious effort to develop new leaders.

_____ B. Training and support are offered to new leaders as well as to more experienced leaders (by our own members or through outside agencies).

_____ C. A "buddy system" matches less experienced members with leaders to help them learn jobs and make contacts.

_____ D. Stakeholder committees are given serious work to do.

_____ E. Leadership responsibilities are shared (e.g., chairing a meeting is a job that rotates).

6. Effectiveness of Your Partnership's Planning and Doing

_____ A. At the beginning of each new year, the effort develops a plan that includes objectives and activities that it wants to accomplish during the year.

_____ B. Plans are based, at least in part, on information collected from surveys of stakeholders.

_____ C. After each activity or project, the leadership or the Coordinating Committee evaluates how things went in order to learn from the experience.

_____ D. We frequently organize visible projects that make a difference to members.

_____ E. When projects are undertaken, action plans that identify tasks, who will do what, and target dates are developed.

7. Your Effort's Use of Research and External Resources

_____ A. The partnership works with other groups in the community on common issues and with citywide organizations that work on critical community concerns.

_____ B. The partnership uses resources and information of other organizations that can help the community (e.g., training workshops on environmental organizing).

_____ C. We stay on top of issues affecting communities across the city and state.

_____ D. Outside speakers come to meetings to speak on topics of interest to stakeholders.

_____ E. Leaders know where to get necessary information (e.g., statistics, forms).

8. Your Partnership's Sense of Community

_____ A. The initiative plans social time at meetings so that people can talk informally and build a sense of community.

_____ B. We plan fun social activities in addition to working meetings.

_____ C. We treat everyone in the group equally.

_____ D. We recognize all contributions, large and small.

_____ E. We make all residents feel welcome regardless of income, race, gender or education level.

9. How Well Your Initiative Meets Needs and Provides Benefits

_____ A. We make resource lists and important contacts available to stakeholders.

_____ B. We hold workshops with "experts" who can provide concrete services to members.

_____ C. As much as possible the effort helps out members with issues of individual need.

_____ D. If a survey of the members indicated that personal issues (such as childcare or landlord-tenant problems) were getting in the way of resident's involvement, the group finds a solution that enables the resident to participate in the organizing of the effort.

_____ E. We hold meetings and workshops where residents can meet elected officials and city service personnel to voice their opinions and learn about resources and programs in the community.

10. The Group's Relationship with the Elected Officials, Institutional Leaders and Other "Power Players"

_____ A. Leaders know how to negotiate with "power players" such as elected officials and institutional leaders and successfully "win" on issues of concern to members.

_____ B. The group has regular representatives who attend important community meetings.

_____ C. All stakeholders understand the lines of authority, decision-making power, responsibilities and other aspects of the "power structure" of the community.

_____ D. The leadership meets regularly with officials about the issues that concern members.

_____ E. The initiative participates in citywide activities and demonstrations that focus on community issues.

DIAGNOSIS SCORE SHEET

Add the scores from A to E together for each section of the Risk Factor Diagnosis. Fill out this score sheet using the total from each section as your total score. The following page will help you evaluate your score.

TOTAL SCORE

1. Vision and Sense of Purpose   _____

2. Effort's Structure   _____

3. Outreach and Communication   _____

4. Meetings   _____

5. Membership Responsibility and Growth   _____

6. Doing Projects   _____

7. Research and External Resources   _____

8. Sense of Community   _____

9. Needs and Benefits   _____

10. Relationship with Power Players   _____

FOR EACH SECTION, FOLLOW THE GUIDELINES BELOW

If you scored between:

5–15	Checkup time! You may need an "overhaul" in this area. Take a look at the Suggestions and Strategies section in the workbook that follows!
15–20	Watch out! It's time for a "tune-up" to get everything in good working order. Look at the Suggestions and Strategies section in the workbook that follows for some ideas.
20–25	Congratulations! You're running smoothly and all systems are go! Keep up the good work! (You may want to read the workbook for some new ideas and inspiration.)

Do you need a complete overhaul of your meetings?

Are you looking for a "tune-up" of your organization or partnership's structure?

Maybe you are running smoothly in the area of vision and goals but hoping for a few pointers?

The following section contains suggestions and strategies for improving all of the areas outlined in the worksheet you have just completed. Depending on your score in each area, you may want to concentrate on specific sections of this workbook.

**SUGGESTIONS
& STRATEGIES**

1. Clarity of Your Vision and Goals

A clear vision and sense of purpose make your initiative proactive instead of reactive, and that means stronger. Outsiders have more respect for an effort with a clear vision and goals, and possible new members will be more willing to join.

Some ways to get the word out on vision and goals are to

- Hold regular orientation or "get to know the effort" meetings for new members at the beginning of each month. Make sure to include an overview of your vision and goals.

- Come up with an attractive flyer that outlines your vision and goals and pass it out at all meetings. This includes meetings with "power players" and other people who are not stakeholders.

- Make a permanent box in the upper right corner of your newsletter that states your vision and goals. This way, even those who don't attend meetings will be aware of where the effort is going and what you want to accomplish.

2. Effectiveness of Your Initiative's Structure

Some key factors contribute to a good organizational structure. These include regular and good meetings, active committees to allow stakeholders to become involved in the issues they care about the most, good by-laws that really represent the effort, and consistent and clear communication among members.

Some things you can do to strengthen the structure of your initiative include the following:

- Have a regular meeting cycle so that stakeholders can anticipate and plan for meetings and new members can easily attend.

- Have written copies of the by-laws available at all meetings, especially the orientation meetings for new members. Explain what they are when you pass them out! Don't just leave it up to stakeholders to figure out the by-laws for themselves. And remember to tell everyone . . . the by-laws change and are updated as the effort progresses.

- Elect or appoint chairpeople of committees to act as "communication central" between the stakeholders and the Coordinating Committee. Have a regular schedule of meetings among stakeholders,

Coordinating Committee and executive board. Don't just leave it up in the air until something "important" comes along.

- Have the Coordinating Committee meet regularly and let stakeholders know when and where the meetings are. This way, members feel they really can talk to the leadership.

3. Effectiveness of Your Outreach and Communication Tools and Methods

Regular communication and input from other residents are the most important parts of a good communication system. Surveys are the best tool for finding out what community residents regularly want and expect from your collaborative effort.

Some ways to do this effectively are to

- Start a newsletter right away! This is a great way to keep everyone informed about your goals and activities and the benefits of joining the effort.

- Survey members and other residents to find out what everyone's key issues and needs are and to create a "buzz" among neighbors that your initiative cares about what residents think.

- Publish survey results in your newsletter and, most important, really use what you learn from the survey to decide on projects and direction. It's not enough to just get the information. YOU HAVE TO USE IT AND LET PEOPLE KNOW YOU ARE USING IT!

4. Effectiveness of Coalition Meetings

If good meetings mean good participation, then bad meetings mean there is a problem! Pay attention to the three areas of meeting management: PLANNING, HOLDING and RUNNING a meeting.

Some key suggestions for good meeting management are as follows:

- Learn to hold effective meetings: Start and end on time, get the agendas out in advance, target members who will be interested in the subject to attend, and never hold a meeting for a meeting's sake.

- Make meeting times and locations convenient: ask "when and where" questions on your survey, and create a volunteer "meeting escort service" if stakeholders are afraid to go to meetings after dark.

- Provide child care at meetings to maximize attendance: ask about childcare needs in your survey. Then hire local teens or seniors.

- Get interpreters of other languages to ensure good participation and LET PEOPLE KNOW IT ON THE MEETING FLIER! Who can interpret? Staff of a local community organization or one of your stakeholders.

- Stick to your agenda and chair with a fair but firm hand! People won't come back if they think your meetings are time wasters.

5. Opportunities for Member Responsibility and Growth

Residents participate in collaborations for many reasons, including having a voice in their community's future and meeting their neighbors. One of the most important benefits members look for, however, is an opportunity to learn new skills and take on personal challenges.

Some ways to give members real opportunities are to

- Create a "buddy system" in which newer "potential" leaders are matched with more experienced members to work in teams for a year so that a real transfer of skills, knowledge and contacts can take place. Advertise this buddy system in your newsletter and at meetings, and you'll probably get more new leaders stepping forward when they know that they will not be left out on their own.

- Look for outside training workshops and conferences that are free or low-cost and send both your experienced and newer leaders. Look for organizations that provide training and workshops for community leaders on organizing and leadership skills. (Check out your local community college.)

- Delegate work wisely and well; if you follow the rules of good delegating, you are bound to develop new leaders and new skills among your stakeholders. Remember:

  ▲ Delegate only one task at a time and make sure it is one that the stakeholder is capable of doing.

  ▲ Be available for questions and provide resources and contacts.

  ▲ Monitor how the job is going; guide but don't interfere.

  ▲ Take time to evaluate how it all went when the job is done.

  ▲ Criticize privately and PRAISE PUBLICLY!

- Give committees decision-making power and real work to do. Don't leave only the busy, boring work for everyone else and keep the important stuff for the leadership. Let committees decide which programs the collaboration will do and make it clear that they can meet with "power players" on their own.

- Try sharing some leadership responsibilities with everyone; for example, chair meetings on a rotating basis among all of the members.

6. Effectiveness of Your Partnership's Planning and Doing

A partnership that plans ahead, in the long and short term, and plans effectively, is respected by stakeholders and nonmembers alike and has the power to really get out and do things! Being proactive means that you plan ahead, and that means projects are effective and successful, one of the best guarantees of great participation!

Some key elements of successful planning are as follows:

- Hold a special meeting at the beginning of each year to develop a plan for the year, including goals and activities and major changes in the community. Make sure you use information you found in surveys of residents about things that they want. Publish it in your newsletter or distribute it separately at meetings.

- Make sure that some of your projects are visible and make a symbolic difference to stakeholders, such as getting a stoplight at a busy intersection or a vacant lot cleaned. Visible victories attract members. Make sure you celebrate and advertise your accomplishments.

- Take project ideas and strategies and break them down into good action plans that identify specific tasks, who is responsible for what, and target dates for getting things done. When you leave it too general, lots of important details fall through the cracks, and your project can backfire. Action plans also give everyone an idea of which jobs need to be carried out and how they fit together.

- Come up with a regular way to monitor all of the jobs. Hold group meetings every two weeks or so to review everyone's progress on their tasks or call everyone separately every week or so to check in on progress and answer questions.

- Make evaluation a regular "wrap-up" activity after projects are finished. Everyone learns from mistakes, and it will give you time to celebrate your successes and praise work well done. Hold an evaluation meeting very soon after every project to go over both process and tasks.

7. Your Effort's Use of Research and External Resources

Knowing when you need outside information and assistance and getting it can be critical for the success of your projects. So can linking up with other coalitions that may be working on similar issues or that may have similar goals. As we have said before, effective projects attract members.

Something to keep in mind about outside resources:

- Look for and work with other coalitions or citywide organizations that are working on similar issues. You can find them by asking local elected officials and community-based organizations and even asking your neighbors. You will learn a lot from working with other groups, and there is strength in numbers.

8. Your Partnership's Sense of Community

One of the biggest benefits residents look for in joining a collaborative effort is a sense of community and belonging. This includes getting to know other residents who may share similar concerns and interests, and feeling like an appreciated and valuable member of the group. A sense of community can be developed in different ways.

Some things you can do to help create a sense of community are as follows:

- Build social time into your meetings so that people can talk informally and get to know each other or catch up on "non-business" issues. A good place for this is before or after the meeting, when refreshments are being served.

- Plan some fun activities! All work and no play makes for a boring partnership anyway! Plan family picnics with plenty of activities for the kids and time to talk informally for the parents, or weekend trips to amusement parks (you can often get great group discounts). You may even want to develop a social committee to plan fun activities.

- Show appreciation for work done! Make a special column in the newsletter that recognizes the "Stakeholder of the Month" for a job well done. Have award dinners at the end of the year where members are appreciated publicly, and give out certificates for even the smallest job as a way of saying thanks.

- Make sure that the effort welcomes all residents, regardless of income, race, gender or education level. You can show this by

  ▲ Having special events that celebrate different cultures, such as Christmas, Channukah and Kwanzaa

  ▲ Holding workshops on issues specific to women and men such as "Being a single father" or "How older women can re-enter the workforce"

  ▲ Making sure that all written materials are read aloud at meetings in case there are members who cannot read

  ▲ Personally welcoming new members either before or after meetings

9. How Well Your Initiative Meets Needs and Provides Benefits

Another reason people join and STAY in a collaborative effort is for the concrete benefits they get. This could involve bringing in an "expert" who speaks about how parents can help their children with homework or how tenants can force their landlord to give them heat and hot water. It could also be something as simple as an introduction to the principal of the school. Your initiative's ability to meet stakeholders' needs and provide a range of benefits is critical for its survival and growth.

Some ways that you can meet needs and provide benefits are as follows:

- Provide members with copies of your lists of contacts with local elected officials, city service agencies, neighborhood institutions, police, and any other contacts and resources. Stakeholders will appreciate them.

- Invite outside speakers to come to meetings and speak on topics of interest to members. Sponsor workshops with "experts" who can provide concrete services to members, such as help with housing problems, entitlement programs, and so on.

- When a member comes to you with a problem, it IS the partnership's problem! Try to help with issues of concern to members. Help set up meetings between a parent and a principal concerning a child, or anything else that the partnership can do.

10. The Group's Relationship with Elected Officials, Institutional Leaders and Other "Power Players"

Having connections to people who "call the shots" in your community is one reason people will join your effort. Being able to negotiate successfully with these folks is a reason people will stay. Regular communication and contact with district "power players" and an understanding of how the "system" works can give you a lot of power.

Some things you should think about doing include the following:

- Learn how to negotiate effectively with "power players" so you can "win" on issues of concern to members. If no one in the partnership knows how to negotiate, send your leaders to a course at a local community college or union.

- Make sure you regularly send a representative to important scheduled meetings. If the same person can go each time, great! When the same person attends meetings consistently, she begins to develop relationships with other regular meeting attenders and can network more effectively.

- Research! Find out how the power structure works so you know who to target for what and who can put pressure on whom. Some of the important questions are

    ▲ What are the lines of authority? Who is whose boss?

    ▲ Who has decision-making power? Over which resources, projects, budget lines, etc.?

    ▲ What is the power structure in the community?

Convening the Community

Identify facilitative, collaborative leadership

Define the scope and parameters of the effort

Develop and implement effective vehicles for two-way communication

Research potential stakeholders

Invite stakeholders

Build the trust and credibility within the stakeholder community

Convening the Community

Critical Success Factors

- Include diverse stakeholders
- Acknowledge the "spark" or catalyst of the process
- Frame both the process and desired outcomes to generate buy-in from all the stakeholders
- Ensure credibility by including visible as well as "non-traditional" leaders

Coordinator and Staff	Coordinating Committee	Stakeholder One	Stakeholder Two	Stakeholder Three	Stakeholder Four
		Step 1 Identify facilitative collaborative leadership • Four buddies who are excited and committed to the idea			
♫	**Step 2** Define the scope and parameters of the initiatives				
	Step 3 Develop and implement effective vehicles for two-way communication • Written documentation of scope and parameters has been agreed on by steering committee. • An outreach and communication committee has devised a communication plan.				
	Step 4 Research potential stakeholders				
♫	**Step 5** Invite stakeholders that reflect the diversity of the community • Have you involved all key partners? • All diversity is represented. • Community map has pins representing all areas. • Partners who have a stake in the outcome.				
♫	**Step 6** Build the trust and credibility within the stakeholder community • Various ideologies are represented.	♫	♫	♫	♫

> ♫ = Step is done by the corresponding partners as well as the initiator

This process was mapped by: Wendy Dickstein, Lucy Fess, Marty Miller, Sharon McLearn, Peggy Parker and Deborah Redwine

Convening the Community

This Core Process describes steps necessary for mobilizing and organizing the community in a collaborative effort to improve health. Sometimes defining the community requires some "out of the box" thinking. The wide array of community sectors (public, private, religious, education, etc.) should all be considered and included to ensure representation of diverse community viewpoints.

According to Leonard Duhl, MD, one of the many challenges in convening the community is the essential "multisectorality" of the effort. "This is chaotic because not only do you have confusion, you have different languages. The languages of medicine and psychiatry are different from the languages of education and economics. So people spend a lot of time getting to know each other." This time must be factored in and, like the rest of the Core Processes, treated as a major priority.

This "multisectorality," albeit difficult to achieve, is worth the effort. When you think creatively about your goals and desired outcomes, your partnership can appeal to all community sectors. Consider economics to be a compelling reason for many. For example, Tom Chapman, former CEO of Greater Southeast Health System, recognizes that a move toward Healthier Communities also makes economic sense for a hospital:

> Working with our trustees and the financial department, we reached the conclusion that we couldn't devote any more than 7 percent of our revenues to free care and still keep the hospital operation profitable. Since we weren't about to start turning people away, we needed to try to correct some of the problems that had propelled us to offer free care in the first place. . . . We now care for the physical, social and mental well-being of our patients. At Greater Southeast, we don't just treat the illnesses that patients bring to us; we try to treat the diseases that are wracking our community—poverty, illiteracy, drugs and violence. . . . Our healthcare costs will continue to skyrocket until we start to deal with these problems. Our hospital does a mirac-

This "multisectorality," albeit difficult to achieve, is worth the effort.

ulous job of keeping very sick fragile infants alive. Yet, most of that incredibly expensive care should be unnecessary. With good nutrition, proper prenatal care, decent housing, and a little bit of education, most deliveries can be low-cost, joyous events.

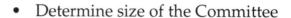

1. Identify facilitative, collaborative leadership.

The initial stage in convening the community is the creation of a Coordinating Committee of community leaders. These individuals not only represent the major interests of the community but have a

"WELCOME TO THE LEADERSHIP SEMINAR. NOW, WILL YOU ALL SIT DOWN AND ALLOW ME TO LEAD THE SEMINAR?"

vision for the community as a whole that goes beyond their own constituency. Together, these individuals catalyze or "spark" the process of collaboration. You should

- Determine size of the Committee

- Agree on leadership and other qualities of effective catalysts

- Identify and meet with potential catalysts

- Gain letters of commitment from each catalyst

- Elect chairs or co-chairs

 While the Initiating (Coordinating) Committee was not a complete representation of the Valley community, it was a diverse enough group to identify potential members for the larger stakeholder group. Almost 400 community members from every possible demographic and economic segment were identified and received invitations to become stakeholders. Of those, over 100 accepted. Over the past year, an additional 100 people have joined the stakeholder group.

— Bill Powanda, Healthy Valley 2000, Derby, Connecticut

Another important consideration for the group is how much to do before all stakeholders are involved:

 It was very important that the Committee not make too many decisions before the stakeholder group formed. The chairperson was selected and the staff was hired but the rest of the organization was not formed until after the stakeholders were selected.

— Deborah Redwine, Oklahoma Commission on Children Youth and P&C Office, Oklahoma City, Oklahoma

☛ *Tip: Build "new" leadership within your effort. Often we see those who lead a collaborative effort feeling overloaded with the responsibilities of committees and projects, on top of the work they are getting paid to do. It usually takes an intentional plan, endorsed by these multirole leaders, to identify and nurture others in the group with interests and abilities for assuming increasing responsibilities within the group. This need is especially great among community groups that have been disenfranchised, where leadership potential has been largely discounted and discouraged: communities of color, women and youth.*

"We had four cities of about equal size (20,000) educated, excited and involved."

— Fran Weisner

2. Define the scope and parameters of the effort.

Once the Coordinating Committee has been established, it agrees on the purpose and scope of the effort. The Committee needs to

- Define the "community" (geographically and otherwise)

- Clarify the costs and benefits of collaboration as a strategy for addressing shared concerns

- Agree on the role of the public (will the effort be "community-wide"?)

- Determine whether to hire a coordinator or other staff (or both) to support the effort

- Determine whether to hire a process facilitator for part or all of the effort

 It was because of this time taken, because of the listening that took place, and because the hospital was willing to let go of the controls, that amazing things happened. The local city and its representatives all said that the project really ought to include the small city community to the north, and then that city said, "Yes, but shouldn't we include the small community to the west?" and so on until we had four cities of about equal size (20,000) educated, excited and involved.

— Fran Weisner, Trinity Hospital, Brookfield, Wisconsin

3. Develop and implement effective vehicles for two-way communication.

The Coordinating Committee is responsible for maintaining clear communication throughout the process. These lines of communication must run throughout the entire community for effective results, using a variety of media to "get the word out." Other suggestions include the following:

- Develop a compelling message and communicate persuasively

- Create an identity or name for the initiative through techniques such as developing a logo

- Take advantage of all connections and relationships within the community

- Air meetings on the local-access TV channel

- Frame the issues, problems and goals of the effort, but leave outcomes open

- Keep the initiative in front of citizens as appropriate (e.g., billboards, radio, newspapers)

- Communicate in all languages of the community (use interpreters, signers)

 A 15-minute presentation of the Healthy Communities philosophy using pictures of local people and activities was developed by the planning committee in October. From November to February, members presented it to 32 different groups, ranging from hundreds of parents at PTOs (Parent-Teacher Organizations) to 20 members of a Saturday morning Masonic breakfast club. Approximately 1,600 people viewed the presentation.

— Peggy Parker, PRO Hampton County, Hampton, South Carolina

4. Research potential stakeholders.

Once the initial purpose and scope of the effort are clarified, the Committee needs to determine who else in the community should be formally included in the process as a stakeholder. Helpful steps within this process include the following:

- Identify and learn how to use stakeholder development tools (such as the Stakeholder Matrix in the Action Worksheets)

"Diversity was evident—from elderly African-Americans who remembered the horse-and-buggy days of Aiken, to high school and elementary students, homemakers and retirees."

— Karen Papouchado

- Agree on the sectors, organizations and constituencies from which representation is needed to ensure the success of the effort

- Identify gaps in representation—stakeholders must reflect the diversity of the community

- Remove or alleviate barriers to participation whenever possible

- Reduce list to those who have time and who will take time

- Consider how stakeholders can be continually added to the effort as needed

 Our diverse stakeholders were recruited in many ways. We found our 300 volunteers through personal contact, church groups, newspaper ads and other means. The volunteers selected themselves into 12 study groups to address the economy, healthcare, education, families, environment, recreation and culture. In addition to 100 volunteers picked by the Steering Committee, over 200 citizens agreed to serve on the study groups for six months. Diversity was evident—from elderly African-Americans who remembered the horse-and-buggy days of Aiken, to high school and elementary students, homemakers and retirees.

— Karen Papouchado, Growing into Life Task Force, Aiken, South Carolina

5. Invite stakeholders.

The Committee, with the assistance of staff, should now develop and send invitations to potential stakeholders. Because no invitation list is ever perfect, it is essential that the Committee move forward even though it may be aware of the need for additional stakeholders from certain interest groups.

- Create an invitation that is clear, compelling and intriguing to a diverse audience

- Develop materials that can be included in the invitation

- Include a faxback form or other means of making it easy to respond

- Create a process for monitoring responses

- Mail invitations

Stakeholder Welcome Letter

Once you have received your RSVPs, send each stakeholder another letter welcoming him or her to your partnership. Include the following information:

1. Location, date and time of the first meeting
2. Current list of stakeholders
3. Draft agenda
4. Reading materials determined by the Coordinating Committee
5. Parking information and maps to the event

Be sure to add any other information relevant to your particular effort.

- Develop a process for personalized follow-up to boost participation
- Develop materials that can be included in the follow-up mailing once RSVP is received (see sidebar)

 Although we began by identifying sectors from which we wanted to ensure representation, we did not explicitly invite stakeholders as representatives. We were concerned that such an identification would box them in, protecting their turf or representing institutional viewpoints. We sought out good personalities for this kind of process, and found that most wore multiple hats. For example, a hospital executive was also outreach chair of an activist religious congregation and a board member of an influential non-profit. We wanted that person to bring all her perspectives to the table.

— Tracy Curts, Greater Dallas Healthy Community, Dallas, Texas

Another interesting point is whom should be seen as the convener:

 Through the Comprehensive Community Health Models of Michigan initiative we have found that using a neutral convener entity (such as a community foundation) has facilitated the process being established within the community as "neutral" and open to all key stakeholders as opposed to having the convening entity being perceived as having its own "agenda."

—Pamela Paul-Shaheen, Comprehensive Community Health Models of Michigan, Battle Creek, Michigan

"We wanted that person to bring all her perspectives to the table. "

— Tracy Curts

6. Build trust and credibility within the stakeholder community.

Throughout the process it is essential that all participants— Committee members, staff and stakeholders—are valued and able to contribute to the best of their ability. It is also important that they begin to see themselves as a group and "critical mass" for change, rather than as a collection of individual interests. A few additional considerations include the following:

- Make each event or meeting flexible, friendly, magical, efficient and effective
- Start and end meetings on time
- Get clear about "why" to collaborate and "so what" if we do
- Make each person feel his or her input is needed

Meetings were always open; anyone could attend and anyone could speak. They always started and ended on time and the agenda was realistic and well planned. . . . The meetings were held at a neutral site, the Community College. The College sponsored breaks and the room meeting space. . . . The meetings were held at the end of the day and ample parking was easily accessible. Food was made available and nametags were large so we could read them from across the room. The room was arranged in a big oval. Microphones were placed for easy access.

— Deborah Redwine, Central Oklahoma 2020, Oklahoma City, Oklahoma

"Meetings were always open; anyone could attend and anyone could speak."

— Deborah Redwine

Your important first step is to assemble a competent team of facilitative leaders, they will be catalysts for further action, . The ideal leaders for a collaborative effort might possess the following attributes:

- Inclusive welcoming stance

- Excellent communication skills

- Conflict resolution skills

- Ability to share the spotlight

- Ability to engender trust among partners

A best-case scenario would be for this group to represent the community on a micro level. Members can be fellow leaders with whom you have worked, or representatives from the community that other leaders have recommended. Above all, make sure this core team is made up of "bridge builders" who can commit a good portion of their time to advancing goals of the coalition. Bridge builders are community leaders who can understand and embrace the goals of your coalition and who can engage other community members in becoming partners in this process.

Defining the scope of the effort and determining the role of the players will be essential. Rather than settling on a limited definition of community, think boldly about all ramifications your effort may potentially have if you involve all sectors and individuals that compose your particular community.

The best ideas on earth will eventually fizzle if they are not communicated appropriately (and later acted upon strategically). Active and effective methods for communication among members of the coalition, and among the coalition and both the community and outside system (e.g., the state), will be vital to the success of your effort. Take advantage of all opportunities available to your partnership for dissemination of your great notions. Use television and radio, create your own newsletter for distribution or to engage the press—leave no communication medium "unturned"! That way, your members, whether they are able to make this month's meeting or not, will all be kept abreast of developments, and your effort will be in the public eye.

Selecting stakeholders is one of the most important tasks before you. The success of your effort depends on engaging the right mix of people. It is not enough to include a handful of prominent, influential citizens who then make decisions for the entire community. Your partnership must be both broad and inclusive, bringing together and working in concert with leaders from all sectors of the community. Ensure that the participants represent a demographic cross section of the community: in age, gender, race or ethnicity, income, education, places of residence, marital status, sexual orientation, language, employment. Don't overlook young people or the elderly, two groups that are often left out of the community change process. They have a great deal to contribute to your effort. Remember, diversity is essential to collaboration. The strength of your effort is really the sum of the capacities of its members. Seeking a broad representation of active members and maintaining an open door are critical to your initiative's success. The Action Worksheets that follow will help you convene your diverse community.

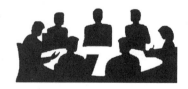

Potential Pitfalls and Strategies

**ACTION
WORKSHEET**

Use the following worksheet as a way to brainstorm solutions for obstacles that might otherwise undermine your efforts.

Potential Pitfalls	Possible Strategies for Bypassing Pitfalls
1. New members and stakeholders are not effectively integrated and oriented.	• Pair new stakeholders with those who have more experience with the effort. • Engage in "ice breakers" before all sessions to help people get to know one another and discuss issues.
2. There is low stakeholder turnout.	
3. There are antagonistic relationships or bad blood among sectors or organizations.	
4. "Usual suspects" lead the process instead of involving emerging leaders.	
5. Coordinating Committee over-committed with its own organizational obligations.	
6. Other Potential Pitfalls . . .	
7.	
8.	

ACTION WORKSHEET

The Community Matrix: Geography, Sectors and Demographics

To ensure that you consider the participation of all community sectors in your effort, use a checklist like the one below.

Geography _____

Sectors	✔ if participant	"I" if individual	"O" if organization
Youth			
Parents			
Local government			
Senior citizens			
Volunteer organizations			
Concerned citizens			
Health services			
Colleges and universities			
School			
Law enforcement			
Faith organizations			
Business			
Transportation			
Community advocate			
Media			
Human resources			
Other. . .			

Used with permission from Micky Roberts, Clarkston Health Collaborative, Decatur, Georgia

The Community Matrix: Geography, Sectors and Demographics *(continued)*

Use the form below to assist you in gathering the information you will need to input into your Community Matrix.

Geography _____

	DEMOGRAPHICS
	We are committed to recruiting a diverse team from our community to participate in this collaborative effort. Please tell us about yourself to assist us in doing this.
Name	
Age	
Ethnicity	
Gender	
Comments	

ACTION WORKSHEET

Inclusivity Checklist

Instructions: Use this Inclusivity Checklist to measure how prepared your effort is for multicultural work, and to identify areas for improvement. Place a check mark in the box next to each statement that applies to your group. If you cannot put a check in the box, this may indicate an area for change.

❏ The leadership of our partnership reflects the ethnic and cultural diversity in our community.

❏ We make special efforts to cultivate new leaders, particularly women and people of color.

❏ Our mission, operations and products reflect the contributions of diverse cultural and social groups.

❏ We are committed to fighting social oppression within the partnership and in our work with the community.

❏ Members of diverse cultural and social groups are full participants in all aspects of our group's work.

❏ Meetings are not dominated by speakers from any one group.

❏ All segments of our community are represented in decision making.

❏ We are sensitive to and aware of different religious and cultural holidays, customs, and recreational and food preferences.

❏ We communicate clearly, and people of different cultures feel comfortable sharing their opinions and participating in meetings.

❏ We prohibit the use of stereotypes and prejudicial comments.

❏ Ethnic, racial and sexual slurs or jokes are not welcome.

Membership

Involvement in your partnership will vary depending on how seriously your effort takes its commitment to empowerment. Consider the following questions with your partnership in mind.

1. How is membership inclusive or exclusive? Who can or cannot join?

2. What, if any, are the financial barriers to membership? For example, does someone have to pay or appeal for scholarships to join?

3. How is membership limited? For example, is the collaborative effort a select group of community leaders with designated posts (e.g., school superintendent, police chief)?

4. How are new members welcomed and oriented to the group?

5. Describe the diversity of the partnership's membership (e.g., geographic, racial, ethnic, economic).

6. Which sectors of the community are represented (educational, religious, business, law enforcement, media, health and human services, neighborhood and citizen groups)?

7. How are explicit attempts made to engage citizens? What role do citizens have in the effort? How is this role stated in the initiative's goals and objectives?

8. At which level(s) and in which ways do citizens and citizen groups actually participate in the collaborative effort?

Collaborative efforts that wish to be successful at accomplishing empowerment goals need to have open and inclusive membership for all citizens; be diverse and multisectoral; and, most important, have citizen and citizen group membership in the partnership.

Stakeholder Selection Guidelines I.

Stakeholders in your partnership should represent the demographic makeup of your community. Use the following guidelines to help you fill in the Stakeholder Selection Chart (which follows the guidelines) and to ensure that you recruit a diverse group.

Major demographic categories to consider:

GENDER
Male—M
Female—F

AGE
Teens—T
Young Adults—YA (born after 1960)
Baby Boomers—BB (born after 1945)
Middle Age—MA
Senior Citizens—SC

PART OF REGION

ETHNICITY
Hispanic—H
Native American—NA
African American—AA
Caucasian—C
Asian—A
Other—O

Other categories to consider:

INCOME
Unemployed—U
Working Poor—WP
Low Income—LI
Middle Income—MI
Upper Income—UP

DIFFERENTLY ABLED
Challenged Mentally—CM
Challenged Physically—CP
Health Challenged—HC

MARTIAL STATUS
Single—S
Married—M
Divorced—D
Widowed (er)—W
Single w/children—SP

RESIDENCY
Established Resident—E
New Resident—N
Part Time—PT
Immigrant Status—IM

EDUCATION
No High School Diploma—N
High School Diploma—HS
College Graduate—CS
Graduate School—GS

SEXUAL ORIENTATION
Heterosexual—H
Lesbian—L
Gay—G

LANGUAGE
Spanish—S
English—E
Other—O

Stakeholder Selection Guidelines II.

The following list should be used for selecting one hundred stake-holders to represent a broad cross section of interests in the community. This number will differ from community to community, but will serve as an example in this case. Individuals selected should be capable of representing the overall interests of the community as well as the interests of the stakeholder group they represent.

Suggested Number	STAKEHOLDER GROUP	Suggested Number	STAKEHOLDER GROUP
20–25	**BUSINESS** Retail Restaurants Agriculture Legal Financial Tourism Industrial Media Transportation Utilities Construction Manufacturing	20–25	**HEALTHCARE** Hospitals Clinics Insurers HMOs Public Health Health Professionals Mental Health Substance Abuse
20–25	**NON-PROFITS** Arts Environmental Human Services Athletics and Recreation Service Orgs. Religious Orgs. Labor Youth and Sr. Services	10–15	**EDUCATION** Child Care Preschool K-12 (Public) K-12 (Private and Parochial) Higher Education Trade and Vocational Adult Education
10–15	**GOVERNMENT** City County State Federal Elected Officials	10	**GRASSROOTS LEADERS** Neighborhood High Risk Youth Senior

ACTION WORKSHEET

Stakeholder Selection Chart

Use this chart to propose stakeholders to be invited to participate in your collaborative effort. Fill out the information on each person to the best of your knowledge, using lists on the previous pages for reference. This will help you pick stakeholders who represent a broad cross section of the community.

Name	Stakeholder Group	District	Gender	Age	Ethnicity	Education

Creating a Shared Vision

Define the scope of the vision

Design the visioning event

Conduct the visioning event

Follow up

Creating a Shared Vision

Critical Success Factors

- Develop the shared vision through consensus
- Distinguish the shared vision from shared values
- Invite all stakeholders to continually re-create and refine their shared vision
- Encourage stakeholders to THINK BIG!

Coordinator and Staff	Coordinating Committee	Stakeholder One	Stakeholder Two	Stakeholder Three	Stakeholder Four
	Step 1 Define the scope of the vision				
♫	**Step 2** Design the visioning effort • Ownership?				
Step 3 Conduct the visioning event	♫	♫	♫	♫	♫
Step 4 Follow up					

♫ = Step is done by the corresponding partners as well as the initiator

This process was mapped by: Tracy Curts, Ivette Rivera Guzman, Reynolds Honold, Kevin Sass, Lynn Shine, Debra Trautman and Julia Weaver

Creating
a Shared Vision

In this Core Process, stakeholders, staff and Coordinating Committee develop a bold, vivid picture of what they would like their community's health to be. A vision that articulates a broad sense of the collaborative effort's common purpose is an essential step and one that is commonly undertaken early in the effort. This establishes the arena in which the partnership wants to work. It is helpful to link your shared vision to community health indicators up front, thereby setting your data-collection boundaries early in the process. For a handful of partnerships, this is a straightforward task. For the vast majority, it is the product of considerable labor and negotiation.

A key guiding principle that has emerged from Peter Senge's work in building learning organizations is the importance of a shared vision. According to Senge:

> A shared vision is not an idea. It is not even an important idea such as freedom. It is, rather, a force in people's hearts, a force of impressive power. It may be inspired by an idea, but once it goes further—if it is compelling enough to acquire the support of more than one person—then it is no longer an abstraction. It is palpable. People begin to see it as if it exists. Few, if any, forces in human affairs are as powerful as the shared vision.

(From *The Fifth Discipline Fieldbook*, ©1990, Bantam Doubleday Dell. Reprinted with permission)

A vision is a compelling statement of what you want to create. It is the engine that drives strategies and gives them force. Once you have a vision, strategies need to be developed to focus your efforts on achieving the vision. But take things one step at a time. The establishment of a shared vision merits careful consideration.

Partnership members must clearly define their shared vision and ensure that identified goals incorporate the self-interests of all stakeholders, plus something larger than those self-interests. Collaboration requires both a realistic understanding that addressing the self-interests of participants is crucial, and a willingness to set aside personal

"Few, if any, forces in human affairs are as powerful as the shared vision."

— Peter Senge

agendas for a common good. Striking a balance between these agendas is critical to your partnership's success.

1. Define the scope of the vision.

The Coordinating Committee should clarify the purpose of a shared vision in achieving its desired outcomes, and develop a process for continually revising the vision. They also need to

- Determine how far into the future they would like to vision
- Link the shared vision to the community's health indicators
- Develop a process for creating a shared vision
- Develop mechanisms to disseminate the vision inside and outside the partnership
- Gain endorsement from major constituencies for the vision development process and scope

 Creating a Healthier Macomb utilized its committee structure to draft the shared vision for health in the community. A subcommittee of the steering committee began the process through fairly traditional methods of developing a vision, including the identification of vision elements and specific definitions for those vision elements. The draft of this vision statement was worked through the steering committee by consensus. That draft was then taken to the community at large and affirmed through a pseudo–focus group process which included presentations and feedback sessions from a wide variety of constituencies in the community including education, business and industry, civic groups, individuals, health care organizations, etc. In all, an estimated 500-plus people had a formal opportunity to review and respond to the draft of the shared vision, which was formally adopted following the affirmation process in the community.

— Scott Adler, Creating a Healthier Macomb, Clinton Township, Michigan

"From the beginning it is essential to create alliances and trust among diverse community segments."

—Kathryn Wilson

2. Design the visioning event.

This can be a staff and Coordinating Committee function. The initial visioning process begins with an event for all stakeholders, early enough in the effort to ensure that the effort is "vision-driven." Visioning can be continued by an Action Team that further develops the vision. In designing the visioning event, staff need to

- Determine the event format and location. The location should be conducive to reflection (green space, garden, glass or open walls).

- Develop an agenda and other packet materials (see sidebar).

- Invite all stakeholders.

- Identify and hire a facilitator and a graphic recorder (use cultural sensitivity when choosing the individuals who will be interacting with your diverse group).

- Purchase materials needed for the event (paper, markers, refreshments, etc.).

- Arrange the room to facilitate dialogue (good acoustics, appropriate size).

- Arrange the room so that new stakeholders interact with more experienced ones.

- Allow enough time for the event (even though there will be revisions).

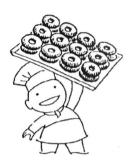

 Remember that people are passionate about "community." From the beginning it is essential to create alliances and trust among diverse community segments. When stakeholders feel threatened by opposing beliefs, they may feel that they will have to "give up" or change their vision of a healthier community. For a diverse group to progress, a skilled facilitator is often necessary—preferably someone who does not have a vested interest in the politics or economics of the community. It should be someone who respects the group process and the underlying concept that the power of the partnership is vested within its membership.

— Kathryn Wilson, Partners for Prevention, San Diego, California

3. Conduct the visioning event.

All stakeholders, staff and Coordinating Committee members participate in the event. To make the most of the event, the facilitator may engage "table facilitators" to assist in ensuring that the event is engaging and yields the

---

Stakeholder Packet Suggestions

- Proposed agenda
- Roster of participants
- List of collaborative efforts currently underway in the community
- Vision statements from other efforts
- Evaluation form

"Our vision has guided us throughout the process."

— Kandiss Bartlett

desired results: a compelling, shared vision of community health. To do so, the facilitators should

- Provide ample tools to allow free expression (written, drawn, etc.)

- Avoid dialogue about strategies (what do we do about the problems?)

- Encourage participants to be bold and embrace contradictions and ambiguity when necessary

- Encourage participants to think 20–25 years into the future

- Focus on common ground; avoid trying to negotiate conflict

- Identify issues or goals that cannot be compromised

- Allow input and feedback, and encourage discussion

- Provide examples of how visions have been used

- Encourage all contributors to join in presenting the group vision.

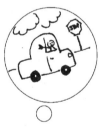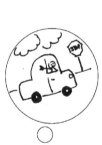 We developed our vision during the full-day retreat. Each individual wrote down her or his personal vision of San Luis Valley Community Connections on a sticky note. We placed them on the wall and grouped them. A writing committee integrated these visions and brought their proposed vision to the larger group, explaining how they selected the wording to represent the personal visions from which it was drawn. The larger group discussed it thoroughly, then agreed upon the final wording that would be presented at the next meeting. At that meeting the vision was amended and accepted in its final form. Our vision as created by the stakeholders is: "San Luis Valley Community Connections creates a responsible, safe, healthy, self-reliant and harmonious community." Our vision has guided us throughout the process, serving as our reference as we discussed the Community Health Profile.

— Kandiss Bartlett, San Luis Valley Community Connections, Alamosa, Colorado

Another good example of conducting the visioning event comes from a group in Palm Springs:

We used the typical "visioning" experience guided by facilitator. The 65 Palm Springs in Action! stakeholders participated in a four-hour "visioning workshop." During the visioning workshop, stakeholders were instructed to visualize Palm Springs in the year 2010 just as they would desire it to be—the Palm Springs of their dreams, in the most optimistic sense. They were asked to visualize how people worked, played, learned; characteristics of governance, the environment, and general aspects of life. Small groups shared their collective ideas with the larger group. The large group then reached a consensus as to the visual images they desired to represent Palm Springs in the year 2010. Those visual images were categorized by general topic. A group of 10 stakeholders volunteered to transform the long lists of images into a more appealing format. Priorities were established to guide the writing of the document. They desired the document to be brief enough to encourage reading, to have emotional appeal, to be general statements so that it would not suggest priorities, and to embody the principles included in the images suggested by the larger stakeholder group.

—Kelley Green, Palm Springs in Action - California Healthy Cities Project, Palm Springs, California

4. Follow-up.

This is an often-overlooked step. To get the most mileage out of the vision, the Coordinating Committee and staff need to ensure that it is linked to the future of the effort. To do so, they need to remind stakeholders regularly of the vision and give them opportunities to continually revise it. The Committee and staff also need to publicize the vision as a way of validating it with the community and increasing the partnership's credibility. Steps include the following:

- Get media coverage of the vision

- Hand off initial vision to an Action Team that will further refine it

- Develop mechanisms for validating the vision with others in the community

- Create opportunities for updating and revising the vision

- Link the vision to all the other phases of the initiative

"Follow-up" is important. It reminds everyone that their accomplishments were important and will provide for further action."

— Lynn Shine

"Follow-up" is important. It reminds everyone that their accomplishments were important and will provide for further action. Create a "media event."

— Lynn Shine, Healthy Communities Index, Durango, Colorado

Communities Alive! focused on creating and circulating a Final Report that detailed their vision:

 An attractive color Final Report of the Community Forum is being sent to all participants, board members of the sponsoring organizations, and will be used as a promotional tool during community presentations. This report contains a three-page reproduction of our community vision, as well as colorful depictions of other activities that happened at the Forum. We feel this report will enable the community to better understand the healthier communities movement and will build interest.

— Lucy Fess, Communities Alive!, Troy, Ohio

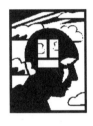 **The following are vision examples from a variety of community initiatives across the country.**

Vision: Roseville, California

The vision established by Roseville Healthy City Coalition states:

"As we serve, we will be guided by the following beliefs:

- That a new vision of health is needed to guide our efforts to enhance the quality of life of our community.

- That the development of the new vision of health is a shared responsibility involving all segments of our community.

- That the new vision of health will evolve through time, as our community periodically redefines its health needs.

- That high levels of ethical and moral values are important components of a healthy community.

- That the dignity and worth of each person in our community deserves respect.

- That health status is impacted by education, income, shelter, safety, sanitation, nutrition, and life-style choices.

- That inequities in health status should be reduced by removing barriers that limit individual potential and well being.

- That the health of the city is an aggregate of individual, family, and neighborhood health."

Vision: Burnsville, Minnesota

The vision from Partnerships for Tomorrow of Burnsville, Minnesota, "was crafted by a collaboration of Burnsville community members and stakeholders (city and county government, business, schools, healthcare organizations, social service agencies and faith communities: We believe in the community of Burnsville. It is a place with a very special quality of life that we must take care to nurture and improve. We believe partnerships between and among the people, schools, governments, churches and community organizations are the best way to ensure that our children's quality of life will exceed our own. We accept a responsibility to plan and implement our vision of the future for that purpose."

Vision: Reno, Nevada

The spirit of the quality-of-life process found its roots in the vision statement of the Truckee Meadow Regional Plan from Reno, Nevada:

Our vision of the Truckee Meadows Region in 2007 is a community where clear views of the mountains from the two cities' downtowns symbolize the economic growth of unique urban centers, surrounded by accessible natural areas and open spaces which support our active outdoor style of life. The Regional Planning Governing Board intends to use planning to achieve this vision, ensuring that regional economic growth continues, based on a mix of traditional and new industries: air quality and other environmental assets are protected; urban sprawl and traffic congestion are reduced; residents are provided choice in housing and employment, in urban and rural settings; and public facilities and services support a high quality of life for all citizens.

Vision: Philadelphia, Pennsylvania

The City Wide Planning and Improvement Agency of North Philadelphia, Pennsylvania, has a very specific vision: "Working together, in collaboration, to create a healthy, supportive environment for the youth of North Philadelphia."

To effect lasting systems change, collaborative partnerships striving toward creating a Healthier Community base priorities on a set of shared values and a clear, compelling vision of an ideal future. Such a force, when translated into a clearly articulated statement of the ideal future, has historically served communities as a guide far beyond the temporal nature of most strategies and plans.

If carefully thought out, a shared vision paves the way for all of the remaining Core Processes, in particular a prioritized action plan. A vision is not a plan, but a shared vision leads to a plan and an implementation strategy that is "owned" by the whole community—one that therefore tends to be self-implementing.

A shared vision also supports the development of long-term, leveraged initiatives rather than short-term fixes and symptom-oriented quick fixes. Addressing what is "broken" does not tend to produce systems change, whereas commitment to the future embraced by a deep, shared vision often does.

Remember, a complex and comprehensive vision takes time and resources. These are both essential ingredients in any collaborative effort. In the words of Creating a Healthier Macomb in Clinton Township, Michigan: "Only by embracing the spirit of collaboration in order to interconnect our endeavors will we successfully achieve our vision."

Potential Pitfalls and Strategies

Use the following worksheet as a way to brainstorm solutions for obstacles that might otherwise undermine your efforts.

Potential Pitfalls	Possible Strategies for Bypassing Pitfalls
1. The vision's scope is defined unrealistically.	• Break down vision components into "doable" segments. • Prioritize vision segments. • Decide on whether you will need to scale down your vision to ensure the scope is realistic.
2. Stakeholders aren't convinced of a vision's importance.	
3. Group has difficulty reaching consensus.	
4. There are logistical complications with visioning event.	
5. Facilitator is seen as an "outsider" who won't understand true community need.	
6. Other Potential Pitfalls. . .	
7.	
8.	

ACTION WORKSHEET

Visioning Dialogue

Arthur T. Himmelman suggests the following exercise as a way to facilitate creating a shared vision:

Before beginning your discussion (about your vision), interview each other for a few minutes in teams of two, by asking your partner the following questions and then reversing the interview:

1. What motivates you to be involved in your collaborative partnership?

2. What do you most want to accomplish through your involvement?

After the interviews, allow time for those who will volunteer to tell the group who they interviewed and what they learned about that person's motivations and hopes. Listen to the reports of these interviews and note the words and phrases that you believe are significant. Using these words and phases, write initial sentences and paragraphs that begin to reflect the vision of your group.

Use this first draft of your vision as the basis for further discussion and refinement by your group.

Reprinted with permission of Arthur T. Himmelman, Himmelman Consulting, Minneapolis.

ACTION WORKSHEET

Creating a Vision

Objective

To help your collaboration create a shared vision or reassess the current vision for future program development.

Procedure

Individually or in a group, write down on a sheet of paper which issue or service is the primary concern of your initiative. For example, if your collaborative effort is primarily concerned with preventing alcohol and other drug use among youths in the community, substance abuse prevention would be your area of concentration. Next, you might consider the following questions.

Discussion Questions

1. What would our partnership look like if we were where we wanted to be in addressing alcohol and other drug use among youths?

2. What would there be more of?

3. What would there be less of?

4. What would be different?

5. Which individual, organizational and community behavior would be different? How would our personal and collective knowledge, attitudes, thoughts and feelings be different?

Now look at the issue that you have listed as primary for your collaborative effort and envision the organization in one year, then five years, by answering the above questions. Discuss your answers. When the group has arrived at a consensus that incorporates everyone's beliefs and values, you have created a shared vision.

From the Southeast Regional Center for Drug-Free Schools and Communities. Reprinted with permission.

ACTION WORKSHEET

Community Visualization

Objective

To help community groups develop a shared vision for a drug-free community.

Procedure

Use the following questions to get people to think about what they want their communities to look like in five years.

Discussion Questions

Visualizing your community in five years . . .

1. What will it be like in your community on a Saturday night in the summer?

2. What will it be like for a child growing up in his or her family?

3. What kinds of things will people say when they talk about the schools in your community?

4. How will the young people in your community view the future?

In a group discussion, individual members of your initiative can share their answers. This process will help you create a shared vision of how your effort can make your community a safe and drug-free environment for youth. The key to creating a shared vision is allowing everyone to have an active role in the process.

From Developmental Research and Programs, Inc.

ACTION WORKSHEET

Visualization

Visualization is another idea-generating exercise that may be helpful for your group. This technique lets people use their imagination to set future goals and actions. If your partnership has been in existence for an extended period, you might want to use visualization to conduct a vision check among key stakeholders.

Objective

To help organizational leadership conduct a vision check among stakeholders.

Procedure

In a group setting, the initiative's leadership or a designated facilitator asks each stakeholder to imagine that he or she is talking with a person that he or she did not know very well. The conversation includes the subject of your initiative and the work that it does. The person says, "Oh yes, I've heard about your collaborative effort. Now what exactly is it that you do?" What will be your response?

Stakeholders are instructed to let their thoughts flow freely and write down the first thoughts that come to mind in the visualization. They can edit their thoughts later.

Discussion

In a group discussion, members share their responses. If some stakeholders have different responses or some have unique answers, then maybe the group has lost sight of the original vision or the partnership has changed so much that members do not have a shared vision. This may be an opportune time for a vision overhaul to ensure that everyone will be committed to the mission and programs of the initiative.

From: Stern, G. J. (1990). *Marketing Workbook for Nonprofit Organizations.* Copyright 1990, Amherst H. Wilder Foundation: St. Paul, Minnesota. Reprinted with permission.

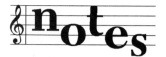

Assessing Current Realities and Trends

Determine who conducts the assessment, and when

Frame the assessment process

Collect secondary data

Map assets

Consider primary data

Inform the public

Collect primary data

Validate and benchmark

Prioritize

Report findings

Assessing Current Realities and Trends

Critical Success Factors

- Measure assets, not just needs or liabilities
- Identify resources that will ensure assessment is effective
- Link assessment to vision, action and outcomes
- Gather relevant and useful information, not just easy-to-find data
- Frame questions from multiple points of view

Coordinator and Staff	Coordinating Committee	Stakeholder One	Stakeholder Two	Stakeholder Three	Stakeholder Four
♫	**Step 1** Determine who conducts the assessment, and when	♫	♫	♫	♫
♫	**Step 2** Frame the assessment process • Scope • Time frames	♫	♫	♫	♫
Step 3 Collect secondary data					
	Step 4 Map assets	♫	♫	♫	♫
♫	**Step 5** Consider primary data • At this juncture either staff or stakeholders may be involved.	♫	♫	♫	♫
	Step 6 Inform the public				
♫	**Step 7** Collect primary data				
♫	**Step 8** Validate and benchmark				
Step 9 Prioritize based on data • Decide whether to go public or remain private	♫				
♫	**Step 10** Report findings				

♫ = Step is done by the corresponding partners as well as the initiator

This process was mapped by: Cheri Fidler, Jim Masterson, Pamela Paul-Shaheen, Ann Solari-Twadell, Connie Williams and Linda Zorn

Assessing Current Realities and Trends

L ike any dynamic entity, your community is the product of numerous factors and influences. To improve the general well-being or any specific element of the community, it is essential to have a clear understanding of the situation. This will also help you monitor progress and evaluate the process and product of your collaboration.

Trends, both positive and negative, should be detected and tracked to help fine-tune community priorities and plan appropriate actions. Given time and resource constraints, your partnership will need to select the most relevant, useful, and accurate measures of assessment. Although there are few absolute standards for indicator selection, following certain guidelines will help you develop the most effective community needs and assets profile. A number of assessment models used by communities across the nation are listed in the Annotated Resources section at the end of the workbook.

Consider the diversity of your community in planning your assessment. Pay particular attention to issues of cultural sensitivity when collecting information from racial or ethnic minority groups, and solicit opinions across the board. The community may be skeptical about your efforts. You will need to do your best to assuage these types of concerns.

Your community's assets must be measured and catalogued as part of your assessment. In this chapter we will introduce the idea of mapping community assets to ensure that you consider all your community has to offer. In Appendix B you will find a Capacity Inventory for your reference.

Assessing current realities and trends includes the steps necessary for gathering accurate, meaningful information about the key dimensions and determinants of health. The assessment should be tailored to the purpose and desired outcomes of the partnership, and create opportunities for insight as well as action by stakeholders, the Committee and the public. It is also a basis for measuring the effect (direct and indirect) of the effort on population health.

1. Determine who conducts the assessment, and when.

Assessment can be used effectively at two stages in the initial effort. (Conducting an assessment at one stage, however, does not preclude conducting one at the other.) Either way, it should be designed and implemented to lead to new insights, awareness and action.

Option 1: Before stakeholders have been convened by the Committee.

In this case, the assessment is conducted by all the Coordinating Committee. The findings are used to spark and inform the subsequent effort.

The Coordinating Committee has collaborated with the Michigan Public Health Institute in the development of a comprehensive community health assessment, and will be working with the CCHMs Evaluation Team in the development of a "Logic Model" for the communities evaluation based on the Logic Model [see Appendix C] created for the project.

— Pamela Paul-Shaheen, CCHMs, Battle Creek, Michigan

Option 2: After the stakeholders have convened and have developed an initial shared vision.

Assessment is a way to understand the gap between vision and reality. The assessment is conducted by stakeholders in an Action Team, and is a bridge to action planning.

2. Frame the assessment process.

All stakeholders involved in the assessment should agree on the scope and time frame of the assessment process. This decision will be influenced by budgetary and human resource constraints. Remember to carefully balance the need for "quick" results against the need for in-depth information. Steps include the following:

• Agree on the purpose and value of assessment in the effort (for both the process and outcomes)

• Determine how the assessment will be "community owned"

- Clarify resources
- Clarify costs and benefits of various assessment approaches
- Decide on the time frame for completing the assessment
- Develop assessment tool
- Determine how the assessment will be linked to action
- Distinguish intended assessment from other assessments in the community

Community participants were involved in the development of the survey as well as the dissemination plan. In this way, ownership was sufficiently established, which enabled us to work with a large group of community volunteers, interns, etc., to go into the community and administer the surveys.

— Micky Roberts, Clarkston Health Collaborative, Clarkston, Georgia

3. Collect secondary data.

Secondary data are sources of information that already exist in a community. Typically, these include a plethora of information in the form of census data; government data from other local, state or federal agencies; and needs assessment findings from health, education, business or other organizations or sectors. They can be documented in various formats, including reports, statistical charts and "white papers." Gathering secondary data should be done early in the effort.

- Agree on purpose and value of secondary data in assessment
- Identify sources of secondary data
- Set limits to the data collection (too much of the wrong information will hinder not help you)
- Collect secondary data
- Identify gaps in secondary data
- Collect data annually

Our collaborative developed a partnership with the Center for Health Information located in the state office of Public Health. Through this partnership we were able to move forward in conducting the most comprehensive assessment within the state of Georgia. The objectives of the project are to assess the health status of the region, identify areas with potential for

> "Community participants were involved in the development of the survey as well as the dissemination plan."
>
> — Micky Roberts

"We are looking at a variety of factors that affect access to health-care and, in turn, health status. These include age, ethnicity, educational level, employment, access to transportation, crime rate, poverty level and other quality of life factors."

— Kevin Sass

change and serve as a catalyst for community health planning. Our approach goes well beyond morbidity and mortality profiles of each life stage or age group. We are looking at a variety of factors that affect access to healthcare and, in turn, health status. These include age, ethnicity, educational level, employment, access to transportation, crime rate, poverty level and other quality of life factors. We are also in the process of conducting inventories of the health and social services available in the counties.

— Kevin Sass, Community Healthcare Network, Columbus, Georgia

4. Map Assets.

Many assessments tend to focus on the needs or problems in a community. Although it is important to identify these concerns, it is equally important to identify the resources, capacities and other assets in a community. These are not just financial but political, economic, social and cultural. All stakeholders should be involved in this process of understanding assets in the community.

- Agree on value and purpose of mapping assets in assessment

- Identify assets or "treasures"

John McKnight and John Kretzmann have written a book on this subject, entitled *Building Communities from the Inside Out: A Path Toward Finding and Mobilizing a Community's Assets*. They suggest how to map the assets of any community and outline the problems using a "deficiency approach," which highlights needs (as opposed to assets) in community development. McKnight and Kretzmann refer to a Capacity Inventory (see Appendix B). They are strong believers that "community development is the process by which local capacities are identified and mobilized," and the Capacity Inventory is their example of a tool to make this happen.

The Capacity Inventory may be tailored to suit the needs of your particular community assessment. The goal, according to the authors, is connecting people with capacities to

- Other people
- Local associations
- Local businesses
- Local institutions
- Capital and credit

5. Consider primary data.

Primary data are data that the Action Team, staff and Coordinating Committee collect themselves. This data should enrich and enliven the understandings gained through the secondary data, and relate directly to the shared vision. If the vision was linked to community health indicators, these indicators should define the data that needs to be gathered. Having reviewed the secondary data, the people involved must determine which primary data should be collected, how and by whom (staff, stakeholders, or both). If they choose to involve stakeholders in data collection, these stakeholders need extensive training to ensure that the data is not "confounded" due to differences in data collection styles.

- Agree on the value and purpose of primary data in assessment
- Determine which primary data are needed
- Identify methods for collecting data (surveys, focus groups, public meetings, etc.)
- Determine who will collect data (staff, stakeholders, or both)
- Develop and provide training as appropriate

6. Inform the public.

At this point the public should be informed that the assessment is underway. Key secondary data that have been collected should be highlighted, and the public needs to be made aware that a process for collecting primary data is about to begin.

- Agree on which findings to highlight and in which formats
- Create a process for responding to any public questions or concerns about the process

7. Collect primary data.

The designated team should now collect actual primary data. Remember to refer to the shared vision for clear indicators of community health to guide the data collection. Too much or irrelevant data will not advance your effort.

- Hold general forums
- Complete observational surveys to document behavior
- Hold community forums

"Community development is the process by which local capacities are identified and mobilized."

— John McKnight and John Kretzmann

- Conduct focus groups
- Conduct household interviews

 Community-based focus groups, as a qualitative research method, allow collection of data concerning health beliefs, attitudes and perceptions. Sixteen focus groups conducted in six different target populations provided an overview of the subjective perspective of both individual and community health in Kent County. The insights shared with the Healthy Kent 2000 Committee by the focus group participants clearly demonstrated the interrelatedness of all aspects of health, and underscored the important role of social, economic and cultural issues in impacting the health of the community.

— Lonnie Barnett, Healthy Kent 2000, Grand Rapids, Michigan

"The insights shared underscored the important role of social, economic and cultural issues in impacting the health of the community."

— Lonnie Barnett

8. Validate and benchmark.

Assessment findings can sometimes be usefully compared to findings from other communities and efforts. When similar indicators exist, findings from these other communities may be used as benchmarks. This enables participants to understand their challenges and assets in terms of the larger context (state, federal, even global). The findings must also be verified and substantiated by the Coordinating Committee, stakeholders and the public.

- Benchmark—compare your findings with those of other communities using the same indicators
- Benchmark with national studies
- Validate with the Coordinating Committee, stakeholders and the public

9. Prioritize.

The Committee and staff review both the primary and secondary data, agree on the most important findings, and organize the data to support priority-setting.

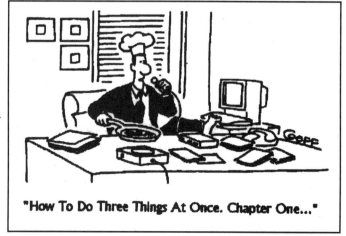

"How To Do Three Things At Once. Chapter One..."

Palm Springs in Action stakeholders spent months studying the realities in our community by (1) developing a Healthy Community Quality of Life Report, (2) using the National Civic League's Civic Index (a self evaluation tool for communities to consider their capacity to work together to solve problems) to evaluate our civic infrastructure and problem solving capacity, and (3) working through a SWOT (Strengths, Weaknesses, Opportunities and Threats) exercise. For selection of key priority areas for improvement, a small group process was used. The entire stakeholder group was divided into four small groups. Each group was assigned to discuss the assessment findings and agree on two priority areas for improvement. All four groups independently chose the same two priority areas: economic development and community safety.

The fact that the choice of priorities was consistent across the groups led the stakeholders to feel the process had been effective and our community successful. Conducting the visioning and assessment steps prior to priority identification ensures priority identification and action plans will be data driven and based on decision-making by consensus.

—Kelley Green, Palm Springs in Action - California Healthy Cities Project, Palm Springs, California

"Conducting the visioning and assessment steps prior to priority identification ensures priority identification and action plans will be data driven and based on decision-making by consensus."

— Kelley Green

10. Report findings.

At this point, the Committee and staff need to determine which findings can be reported to the general public. Once this is determined, they agree on the best methods for publicizing the findings.

- Agree on key findings
- Determine the most effective format for describing the findings— make an impact!
- Determine whether different formats are needed for different uses or audiences
- Agree on which information is "confidential" (for the stakeholders or Committee only)
- Develop and write a report
- Disseminate the report

A whole-person health assessment tool is used to give the individual a baseline perspective of his or her current health. In addition, a group report is generated, which gives the areas of risk of the whole group. The information is then used for structuring the effort.

— Ann Solari Twadell, Advocate Health Care, Park Ridge, Illinois

The process of assessing current realities and trends involves information collection and analysis. It addresses the root concerns of the community by asking specific questions and taking action accordingly.

A good assessment will help your partnership answer important questions, such as:

- What are our community's assets?

- How can we achieve our goals?

- Which existing data are relevant to our effort?

- How far-reaching do we want our results to be?

- What are the obstacles to our progress?

- What are realistic outcomes of our effort?

By assessing current realities and trends, your partnership should gather accurate, meaningful information about the key dimensions and determinants of health. Most likely, your visioning process began this step for you as you linked your vision to the desired health indicators in your community. The assessment should be tailored to the purpose and desired outcomes of the partnership, and should create opportunities for insight as well as action by stakeholders, the Committee and the public. If done thoroughly, it should also link the assessment process to visioning, action planning and outcomes so that continuity is maintained throughout the process.

Potential Pitfalls and Strategies

Use the following worksheet as a way to brainstorm solutions for obstacles that might otherwise undermine your efforts.

Potential Pitfalls	Possible Strategies for Bypassing Pitfalls
1. Focus on deficit vs. asset-based approach to community development.	Use the Capacity Inventory in Appendix B to assist the group in seeing your community's resources as assets.
2. Assessment not specific enough in its questions.	
3. Secondary data available are insufficient.	
4. Few benchmarks exist for the specific community needs your effort has identified.	
5. Findings organized unclearly.	
6. Other Potential Pitfalls . . .	
7.	
8.	

ACTION WORKSHEET

Organize Your Member Skills, Resources and Contacts

Consider the wealth of resources within your own community before launching your external assessment.

List the skills, resources and contacts of your group's members and potential members.

Member Name and Information	Skills, Resources and Contacts

Keeping Track of Community Resources and Institutions

List the institutions and resources in your community. They may become important partners in your work.

Institution	Contact/Address/Phone	Services, Programs

**ACTION
WORKSHEET**

Assessment Distribution

Use this template to create a strategy for distributing your initiative's assessment tool. Add your ideas for outreach strategies in your own community.

Outreach Strategy	Locations and Sites	Volunteers	When?
DOOR-TO-DOOR			
DISTRIBUTING AT MEETING			
SET UP TABLES AT BUSY PLACES (e.g., supermarket sidewalks) TO DISTRIBUTE			
WORKING WITH OTHER LEADERS			

Action Planning

Define the purpose of an action plan

Develop a framework

Conduct design meetings to create the action plan

Write the initial action plan

Validate and revise the action plan

Disseminate the action plan

Action Planning

Critical Success Factors

- Ensure that actions are strategic and leverage-based
- Facilitate ownership by clarifying realistic roles and responsibilities
- Include ambitious and longer-term actions as well as short-term "small wins"
- Define actions in terms of specific and detailed tasks, tactics and objectives
- Anticipate and plan for training and resources

Coordinator and Staff	Coordinating Committee	Stakeholder One	Stakeholder Two	Stakeholder Three	Stakeholder Four
	Step 1 Define the purpose of an action plan				
♫	**Step 2** Develop a framework				
♫	**Step 3** Conduct design meetings to create the action plan	♫	♫	♫	♫
Step 4 Write the initial action plan					
♫	**Step 5** Validate and revise the action plan	♫	♫	♫	♫
♫	**Step 6** Disseminate the action plan				

♫ = Step is done by the corresponding partners as well as the initiator

This process was mapped by: Kurt Kazanowski, Marilyn King, Paul Robertus, Barbara Strack, Mary Lou Stubbs and Eduardo Vasquez Valdes

Action Planning

In this Core Process, the Coordinating Committee—with input from stakeholders and staff—develops and documents a coherent, user-friendly action plan. The plan describes the partnership's goals for improving health, its objectives, and the high-leverage strategies and methods that it will use to address these goals and objectives. It may contain programs, initiatives and projects. The plan assigns Committee members, staff and stakeholders to each goal or program, and defines the time frame for action. Most important, the plan describes how programs and projects will be linked synergistically for most efficient action.

Throughout the plan's development process, special attention should be given to the validation and revision stages, using reactions from stakeholders as well as individuals outside of the effort (e.g., clients and customers) as archetypes of how the community at large will respond to your partnership's efforts. Time spent here is a wise investment in your effort's future and sustainability. The incorporation of changes and improvements at this stage will save time and resources down the road. In your quest for improvement, consider that you will need to evaluate the entire effort at some point; that evaluation device will serve you best if it is developed early in the process (see chapter on monitoring and adjusting for additional information). Above all, remember that there is no substitute for stakeholder ownership of the plan.

A strategic action plan should embody the overarching logic for realizing the original shared vision. If done well, the plan should address identification and deployment of resources in a reasonable time frame as well as detail the impact of the plan on the external environment.

▼

1. Define the purpose of an action plan.

By the time the partnership begins action planning, it can draw on its initial shared vision for health in the community. As it did before creating the shared vision, the Committee needs to agree on the purpose of the action plan and its value in achieving the partnership's vision. The Committee also needs to determine how the action plan can be refined and updated annually (or more frequently). Steps include the following:

- Agree on the purpose and value of an action plan

- Benchmark other types of plans (program, strategic and organizational)

- Link the action plan to other Core Processes, including creating a shared vision and doing the job

- Link the action plan to "community indicators"—to better determine exactly what needs to be done

 Partners for Prevention used the following criteria to choose projects and develop an action plan: (1) It is workable; (2) Requires collaboration; (3) Maximizes existing resources; (4) It is unique; (5) It is needed; (6) It is aligned with the goals of Partners; and (7) It is economically feasible.

— Kathryn Wilson, Partners for Prevention, San Diego, California

2. Develop a framework.

There are a variety of formats for developing action plans, many of which have emerged from strategic and organizational planning. The framework for the partnership's action plan needs to be multiorganizational and multisectoral, and intended to inspire action (not just awareness); it should call for changes in both the short and long terms. At this stage, the Committee should

- Review action plans from other partnerships to see if lessons can be learned from them

- Agree on the level of detail of the plan

- Agree on the time frame of the plan (three to five years is recommended)

- Consider using software programs currently available that assist with action planning (see United Way's COMPASS information in Annotated Resources, page 215)

- Develop mechanisms for ensuring that the plan is linked to actions

- Develop mechanisms for ensuring that the plan is understandable and usable by the partnership itself as well as by the public and other interested parties

- Determine who will develop the plan

- Create a mechanism for revising the plan annually or more frequently

- Identify vehicles for using the plan to continually mobilize action (e.g., "Issue Updates")

- Clarify how to increase accountability and address lack of accountability (stakeholders who don't fulfill their commitment to the plan)

 Planning is often seen as a "one-shot" deal, required at the time to satisfy political needs to "do something." However, in this case, the development of the plan represented only the beginning of the project, with the plan also serving as a contract between participants which states what each will do to address AIDS.

— Patrick Lenihan, Chicago Department of Public Health, Chicago, Illinois

3. Conduct design meetings to create the action plan.

These meetings should include the Committee, staff and stakeholders. The purpose of the meetings is to complete the design of the action plan, using the shared vision and assessment as guideposts. The plan also needs to reflect the partnership's principles and values. Some steps include the following:

- Provide preparatory materials to each participant before meetings (assessment data, etc.)

- Hold meetings with potential clients or customers to gain input on goals and strategies for each program or initiative

- Identify a facilitator who can ensure high-quality group work

- Post partnership information (organizational structure, vision) on the meeting walls for easy reference

- Provide templates and matrixes for organizing complex ideas into objectives and tasks

- Select goals, objectives, strategies and methods

- Agree on budget

- Assign roles and responsibilities

- Ensure that the plan builds on assets

- Consider unanticipated negative outcomes and revise the plan as needed

- Consider how action plan document can show how it is linked to other Core Processes

 Be prepared to address the different sets of "needs" and "assets" that groups with different life experiences will have. One quick example—elderly residents of a minority neighborhood said that streetlights were the top priority in their neighborhood. From local government's perspective, fear reduction (crime watch, etc.) was the "real" issue and resources would be better spent on that than on expensive streetlights. A compromise was crafted so that community-oriented police were assigned to these neighborhoods and had the authority to request streetlights in spots they judged a hazard.

— Karen Papouchado, Growing Into Life, Aiken, South Carolina

4. Write the initial action plan.

This has typically been a staff function but should not be limited if stakeholders want to participate. To make sure the plan is user-friendly, it should use verbs and energizing language as much as possible, and should be presented in an easy-to-understand format. Diagrams and charts outlining time lines and responsibilities are also helpful. Keep in mind that a good action plan can also serve as the basis for future grant applications (for more information, see the Foundation Center reference in the Annotated Resources).

5. Validate and revise the action plan.

The Committee, with staff assistance, should gain the commitment of stakeholders to fulfilling their roles and responsibilities as outlined in the plan. The plan must be verified or determined feasible by all members. Stakeholders must also be given an opportunity to revise the content and format. Steps include the following:

- Identify vehicles for gaining information and ideas: focus groups, phone surveys, gatherings of the whole partnership

---

Sample Agenda for an Action Planning Meeting

Instructions: The best results for action planning will probably come from a meeting in which the facilitator guides the group through the prescribed steps.

A few tips:

- Build breaks into the meeting agenda if necessary (e.g., 15-minute break if meeting exceeds two hours).
- Establish clear time frames for the whole meeting and for each item on the agenda.
- Don't limit discussion too much. People need to feel that their ideas and insights have been included and heard.

Action Planning Meeting Agenda

1. Welcome and introductions
2. Overview of the action planning framework
3. Identifying problems and issues
4. Action planning teams: developing strategies and programs
5. Team reports: what has been developed and discussion of adjustments when needed
6. Establishing the final action plan: tasks, assignments and time frames
7. Getting agreement on the plan
8. Wrap-up: summary of decisions and accomplishments, next steps

---

- Document any and all suggestions

- Agree on how suggestions that are not reflected in the plan should be addressed

- Gain formal commitments by staff, Committee and stakeholders to their roles and responsibilities

- Identify criteria to be considered in reviewing the draft plan

- Revise the action plan

 The constituency groups reviewed the action plan for practicality, useability, asset mapping feasibility, etc. We also had mini focus groups with people or constituency members who also represented other community organizations.

— Kurt Kazanowski, Creating a Healthier Macomb, Clinton Township, Michigan

6. Disseminate the action plan.

The action plan is most likely to lead to action if all stakeholders receive a copy of the plan in a timely manner. It should also be shared with the public and other organizations that may be potential collaborators. Staff should

- Send the action plan—with a cover letter from the Committee—to all stakeholders

- Develop a media packet and dissemination plan

- Organize meetings with all stakeholders to formally confirm their roles and responsibilities

- Send the plan to current or potential collaborators and arrange meetings to confirm their role

- Hold a general or partnership forum to present the plan

> *Tip: You've got to be specific about what you ask and want people to do. For example, we went to the Kiwanis Club, gave them an overview of our project, got them all excited, and then just stopped. They were eager to be of assistance, but we didn't tell them how they might do this, or query them. We didn't ask them for anything tangible, or if they could contribute to any goals. You need to ask, "Would you adopt this goal in your efforts over the next year?"*
>
> — Kurt Kazanowski, Creating a Healthier Macomb, Clinton Township, Michigan

"The constituency groups reviewed the action plan for practicality, useability, asset mapping feasibility, etc."

— Kurt Kazanowski

Strategies are high-level, integrated sets of actions you will take to achieve your vision. From strategies, a tactical or operational action plan is developed that explicitly identifies the scheme of action that people will take to realize the vision.

The action plan is a relatively straightforward task but one that must involve a variety of elements:

- Laying out specific action steps to implement the strategy

- Identifying specific individual stakeholders or stakeholder work groups who agree to be responsible for each action

- Setting time frames for each tasks completion

- Taking into account the multisectoral aspect of the collaboration and ensuring that it is a call to action

The writing, validating and revising of the action plan must be undertaken to provide your effort with a clear understanding of your next steps. Pay particular attention to client-customer and community responses and strive to incorporate changes and use constructive criticism to your benefit—now is the time. Thorough dissemination is vital and will be your best call to action.

Potential Pitfalls and Strategies

Use the following worksheet as a way to brainstorm solutions for obstacles which might otherwise undermine your efforts.

Potential Pitfalls	Possible Strategies for Bypassing Pitfalls
1. Action plan is unclear, unrealistic, "un-action" oriented and overwhelming.	• Contact agencies in nearby communities for suggestions of skilled facilitators whose services might be contributed to assist the group in the refinement of the action plan. • Break the plan down into more manageable tasks and timelines. • Use the Action Worksheets in this chapter to break the action plan into activity, person responsible, resources needed and timeline.
2. Several stakeholders are upset at not receiving updated action plan.	
3. Logistical problems arise at the Design Meeting.	
4. The action plan is not clearly written.	
5. Planners have difficulties agreeing on a budget.	
6. Other Potential Pitfalls . . .	
7.	
8.	

ACTION WORKSHEET

Action Plan Brainstorm

This exercise might be useful for generating ideas for your action plan.

Step 1

Which actions can we take to improve community well-being? Consider new programs or commitments or policies that you believe could have significant results.

Action	Expected Results

Step 2

Now look back at your ideas for Actions. Do we have the capacity to do all these? Which ones are most important to do first? How should we decide which actions to take?

Action Plan Framework

This template may be used as a sample to develop your action plan framework. Keep in mind that your personal effort may call for specifics not detailed in the worksheet below. Use this as a point of departure to create your own customized action plan.

Organization name _____ Date plan completed _____

Activity Description (what is to be done)	Person(s) Responsible	Resources Needed (check on availability)	Time Line*	Comments

*by 6-month increments, e.g.: 6 mo, 1 yr, or 1½, 2, 2½, 3, 3½ years

Points to consider:

- How will this action plan be linked to the remaining Core Processes?

- Which methods will your partnership use to ensure the regular revision of this action plan?

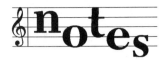

Doing the Job

Capitalize on strengths

Find more partners

Get buy-in

Get and maintain resources

Get the word out

Undertake the projects and initiatives

Deliver the "goods"

Sustain the purpose of the people

Stay focused and fine-tune

Doing the Job

Critical Success Factors

- Link "doing" with vision, assessment, action planning, and outcomes
- Time and link actions so that they are synergistic and systemic
- Balance attention to both short- and long-term actions
- Anticipate and address obstacles
- Capitalize on financial incentives such as pooled funding

Coordinator and Staff	Coordinating Committee	Stakeholder One	Stakeholder Two	Stakeholder Three	Stakeholder Four
♪	**Step 1** Capitalize on strengths • Assets identified • Bridge to action planning	♪	♫	♫	♫
♪	**Step 2** Find more partners				
♪	**Step 3** Get buy-in	♫	♫	♫	♫
♪	**Step 4** Get and maintain resources				
♪	**Step 5** Get the word out • More participation • Positive press coverage • More phone calls coming in				
♪	**Step 6** Undertake the projects and initiatives				
♪	**Step 7** Deliver the "goods" • Are things happening to the degree of satisfaction? • More participation and involvement • Programs being done • Can see some change happening	♪	♫	♫	♫
♪	**Step 8** Sustain the purpose of the people	♪	♫	♫	♫
♪	**Step 9** Stay focused and fine-tune				

♫ = Step is done by the corresponding partners as well as the initiator

This process was mapped by: Dan Baumgarten, Carl Ellison, Mary Hood, Colin Laird, Marilou McPhedran, Patsy Methany, and Marcia Turner

Doing the Job

This is the implementation phase of the effort. The partnership should be "strategic" in how it carries out the initiatives and projects specified in the action plan. Because conditions change—often dramatically—after the action plan is developed, projects are timed, linked, coordinated and ultimately rolled out so they capitalize on political, economic and social resources, and other opportunities. Keep in mind, however, that the feasibility of the action plan must be continually monitored, as these same changing conditions can cause problems and the depletion of resources. The steps in this Core Process are circular, and they overlap synergistically.

In the doing the job phase, collaboration enhances all actions. Not only must the partnership use its internal resources wisely to ensure that all members maximize their personal capacities, but human (and other) resources outside the effort must be considered as potential assets as well. As collaboration is defined as "the exchange of information, the sharing of resources and the enhancement of another's capacity for mutual benefit and to achieve a common purpose," it is incumbent upon your members to clearly communicate this mutual benefit to potential partners.

An essential point to consider is balancing short- and long-term actions with fluidity. While capitalizing on our strengths, we must also be savvy conservationists of our resources. Although short- and long-term actions may appear as separate entities, note overlap and take advantage of progress that may propel you to the next level with less initial investment. This flow between short- and long-term actions, doing the job and action planning, organizing the effort and the remaining Core Processes, illustrates the synergy between any and all components of a true collaboration.

"Each time a person uses his or her capacity, the community is stronger and the person more powerful."
— John McKnight and John Kretzmann

1. Capitalize on strengths.

The Committee and others involved in doing the job review the action plan and ensure that intended projects and initiatives build on the partnership's human and financial assets. Most important, it is essential that this phase include all stakeholders—not simply the Committee—and that the actions are well timed. Steps include the following:

• Adjust and reaffirm consensus on the action plan

• Check for inclusiveness

• Confirm who is doing what

• Make changes in the plan as necessary (to reflect new stakeholders or resources)

• Confirm which skills and resources each individual can bring

In the words of John McKnight and John Kretzmann: "Each time a person uses his or her capacity, the community is stronger and the person more powerful. That is why strong communities are basically places where the capacities of local residents are identified, valued and used. Weak communities are places that fail, for whatever reason, to mobilize the skills, capacities and talents of their residents or members."

Another strong point of your partnership should be how you time your efforts:

Using the action plan as a guideline, we take actions that are timed and coordinated so that they yield the greatest returns.

— Pamela Paul-Shaheen, Comprehensive Community Health Models of Michigan, Battle Creek, Michigan

2. Find more partners.

Although the number and type of partners depend on the scope of the project, the Committee and Action Team will undoubtedly find that there is a need for more partners to ensure a "critical mass" to make the project succeed and to sustain it. They need to

• Identify major collaborations and other potential partners

- List groups that care about the issue, assess their degree of connection to the issue (on a scale of 1–5), and determine whether there is a place for their participation

- Strengthen connection with priority groups

- Look at what is already going on regarding this issue and plan how to "piggy-back" as much as possible

- Anticipate resistance to sharing and build strategy to keep at it

- Invite people's involvement

- Continue to build momentum

- Continue to leverage relationships

 To ascertain interest from diverse stakeholders, a personal visit was made to each agency's C.E.O. and/or Community Services officer, to outline the concept of a coalition of private and public service agencies, business and industry and concerned individuals joining together to address the health and social needs of the community. Upon finding that there was an interest, a meeting was convened in May 1993, hosted by Union Hospital at its off-campus Community Services Building, to form the Township of Union Network with more than 27 charter entities agreeing to participate. Mr. Ted Hardgrove, President of New Brunswick Tomorrow, was the keynote speaker, underscoring what a collaborative approach can accomplish, using his experience leading such an effort in New Brunswick, N.J., as an example.

—Reverend James Roberts, Township of Union Network, Inc., Union, New Jersey

Regarding "Collaborative Empowerment," Arthur T. Himmelmen points out:

> Negotiations with outside agencies and institutions produce agreements to proceed on a collaborative basis based on the collaborative's mission established by the community, and within a governance and administrative process in which power is equally shared by the community and outside organizations.

3. Get buy-in.

Even in partnerships that include all of the key community leaders, there are sometimes other organizations or individuals who have a stake in the outcome but are not formal participants in the effort.

Before implementing a project, it is essential to win the support of those who may not have been engaged earlier on in the effort—especially those who may cast stones at the project or the effort as a whole. Steps should be taken to

- Get and document support from community leaders

- Get and document approval from the governing boards of key organizations

- Meet with "powers that be"

> Getting buy-in started with one person going around interviewing various people from various service organizations for a directory that was being developed. In the interviews the person also asked, "What do you think is needed?" Although we had an idea what we wanted, we had to ask what others wanted, which in our case was simply a framework for getting together on a regular basis to share information and resources among human services organizations.
>
> There are two levels to "getting buy-in": one is to first get people to say yes to actually supporting the effort; and the second, perhaps a little further down the road, is getting people to spend the time and effort to understand each other better before creating partnerships and relationships.
>
> — Colin Laird, Healthy Mountain Communities, Basalt, Colorado

"You don't have a good chance of success if you force an initiative onto a community."

— Mary Hood

At Mercy Mobile Health Care in Atlanta they take a very practical approach to getting buy-in:

> You don't have a good chance of success if you force an initiative onto a community. If a community doesn't believe they have a need or opportunity of which they want to take advantage, then they won't take part. You really need to listen to what the community wants. If we can't help with what they want, then we suggest other partnerships.
>
> — Mary Hood, Mercy Mobile Health Care, Atlanta, Georgia

4. Get and maintain resources.

Resources—financial and other—are the focus of those charged with organizing the effort, but also should be considered in doing the job. Before projects are launched, the Committee staff and stakeholders need to ensure that funding is in place, and should be able to take other actions if resources have not been provided as hoped. They need to

- Identify internal assets
- Commit and coordinate the initiative's resources
- Seek and generate external resources

> We gathered resources only for the initiating stage and the stakeholder selection stage of the process. We sought a lot of our resources during the "get buy-in" stage, in the meetings with organizations and individuals, where we'd ask, "Will you support us and contribute funds/resources?"
>
> — Patsy Methany, Office of Community Partnerships, Columbus, Ohio

5. Get the word out.

Promotion is another dimension of doing the job, which overlaps with organizing the effort. Steps include the following:

- Engage citizen's imagination and excitement (media strategy)
- Orchestrate an "announcement" or "action" kick-off to emphasize goals and acknowledge contributors
- Invite any and all interested parties to the event
- Get the word out through presentations, public meetings and newspaper articles
- Communicate citizens' successes in improving community health
- Keep funders informed (articles, newsletters)

> The Outreach/Public Relations Support Team of the Coordinating Team is establishing a Communities Alive! Speakers Bureau, which will offer presentations to local groups and organizations. These programs will be presented by community volunteers who are working on the Support Team.
>
> — Lucy Fess, Communities Alive!, Troy, Ohio

The following are programs and methods used by The Wellness Centre of Surrey, British Columbia, Canada to "get the word out" to their community:

"Establish a speakers bureau which will offer presentations to local groups and organizations."

— Lucy Fess

- Senior's Planning Committee for delivery of outreach programs
- White Rock Social Planning Committee for a direct line to office of the mayor
- Diabetes Education Program expanded
- Seniors' Substance Awareness Program expanded

— Dolores Kilpatrick, The Wellness Centre, Surrey, B.C., Canada

The Office of Community Partnerships in Columbus, Ohio, also used some creative ideas to broadcast their information:

We used a series of community, individual and mini-group meetings to coordinate the following: billboards, 1-800 call-in lines, flyers, door hangers, newsletters to a mailing list of 5,000, flyers in the water bills, call-in shows on TV and radio talk shows, articles in suburban and main newspapers. We also taped all the stakeholder meetings and showed them on the local TV channel. All this media was coordinated by a paid part-time staff person.

— Patsy Methany, Office of Community Partnerships, Columbus, Ohio

6. Undertake the projects and initiatives.

Before the "goods" are delivered, a good deal of pre-launch work and preparation is done. This can include

- Holding meetings with client-customers and staff of planned programs
- Addressing any last-minute problems in the project or initiative
- Ensuring that funding and other resources are still available

We called our initiative "10,000 Discoveries"; with each "discovery" being a step toward improving health that can occur anywhere, whether through a state congressional effort or a small neighborhood project. Local examples include an effort to improve bicycle safety and another to establish an eligibility program for processing a basic state health insurance plan.

Our approach was to train citizens as "discoverers"; we as an organization merely acted as facilitating catalysts. Citizen "discoverers" take part in a four hour training session in the basic

"We also taped all the stakeholder meetings and showed them on the local TV channel."

— Patsy Methany

skills and support necessary for creating a framework for their effort. We assist them by helping them to set up the basic infrastructure to support their "discovery." We do this by providing assessment advice and by acting as "support brokers," whose purpose is to farm out to the community—or "broker"—support for the initiatives. Health Improvement Partnership helps to make the necessary connections, and then we get out of the way of the "discoverers" or citizens leading the effort. Our approach is designed to stretch people's efforts.

What works best is defining ourselves as catalyst and behaving as such. Our aim is to strengthen people's capacity to do their work, and in the process we become their collaborators and friends. This approach helps to break down barriers and create linkages, and therefore create support.

—Dan Baumgarten, Health Improvement Partnership, Spokane, Washington

> "Our aim is to strengthen people's capacity to do their work, and in the process we become their collaborators and friends."
>
> — Dan Baumgarten

7. Deliver the "goods."

In this step, the projects and initiatives are begun. The collaboration will witness some fruits of its labor, but must also remain vigilant. Important considerations include the following:

- Capitalize on the visibility of this accomplishment to recognize and celebrate hard work

- Ensure that participation remains active after the "goods" are delivered

- Remain aware of quality and not just the delivery of quantity

8. Sustain the purpose of the people.

Once projects begin, it is important to monitor the impact of the actions on the partnership itself. This is another "checkpoint," which includes the following:

- Monitor internal staff: How are we?

- Ensure that the effort is gaining, not losing, strength

- Create identity for the initiative apart from any of its activities or projects

- Have advisory committee's agreement as to monitoring, adjusting and guiding initiative

- Support people in their activities (assessment strategies)
- Energize the coalition through activities
- Increase membership
- Listen to each other

Since late 1994, Healthy Community, Healthy Economy has had an Executive Director to provide staff support focusing. Simple support tactics, such as circulating minutes of decisions made, sending meeting reminders, and preparing tight agendas are helpful. At times, staff have presented options or position papers to speed the process. If necessary, the Executive Director can raise process issues with chairpeople or encourage group analysis of focus problems. In one instance in which focus was an ongoing problem, it was necessary to reformulate the team and provide clearer Board direction.

— Laurel Hayler, Silicon Valley Joint Venture, San Jose, California

"You don't sustain people's purpose; they do. You support their purpose by believing in them."

— Dan Baumgarten

Health Improvement Partnership looks to the people to sustain their own purpose:

Sustaining the purpose of the people comes from believing in people's capacity and always supporting that belief. Start from believing—claiming—that it's possible. Always work toward strengthening people, to what is possible, and to supporting the possibility. You don't sustain people's purpose; they do. You support their purpose by believing in them.

For example, we were working with service managers of an agency that deals with child abuse and neglect. Everyone was overwhelmed, demoralized, unable to maintain the tremendous workload. We brought these overwhelmed managers together and had a trained facilitator ask the group to look beyond their valid personal complaints and gripes and to instead look for a higher goal, purpose, and meaning, one which would better frame the problem and that would make others aware of the problem while motivating them to help. And it worked. The problem of the tremendous workload was framed in regard to how it was an obstacle in providing abused and neglected children the care and support they needed; with everyone focused on helping the children by better helping each other, we

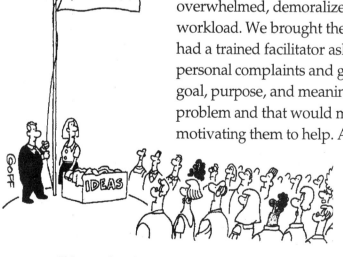

"No one's saluting. Run up another one."

were able to use the group's collective purpose as a point of break-through. Invest in people's capacity to solve problems.

— Dan Baumgarten, Health Improvement Partnership, Spokane, Washington

> ☞ *Tip: Watch for warning signs and conditions that cause nega-tive repercussions throughout the internal members of the part-nership. It is not unusual to be so focused on your goals and objectives that staff is overlooked. Common difficulties include*
>
> - *Tension caused by strained group dynamics, "turfism," leadership, etc.*
> - *Burnout, turnover or other membership and participation concerns*
> - *Top-heavy focus on long term without allowing for short-term successes and celebrations*
> - *Ineffectiveness in achieving desired results due to inadequate planning or resources*
> - *Changes in community situation that dictate changes in vision*

9. Stay focused and fine-tune.

Because it is impossible to predict how a program will be received until it is initiated, the Committee and staff need to make mid-course adjustments based on a variety of data. They may also need to make fairly significant changes in methods, strategies and target audiences to achieve the intended outcomes. They should

- Develop common parameters as start points for program development
- Build on prior assessments and priorities
- Listen to needs and reactions
- Learn more about the problem
- Observe what people are doing
- Review the plan against research data, community input
- Reframe the plan so participants remember vision, goals, tasks at hand

Mercy Mobile Health Care provides a good example of how to review and reframe the plan to maximize efficiency:

 Every year goals for the program are established. The founda-tion has a comprehensive health plan that identifies the priority needs to be met within the two key areas of family health and infectious diseases. Each goal must be related first to values and then to five dimensions of primary care: access, integration, accountability, holistic collaboration and partnership. Presently standards and indicators are also being developed for faith-based partnerships. Allocation of resources is prioritized according to severity of need, potential for long-term impact, prospect of sustainability, and availability of collaborators, funders and human resources. Any new initiative costing more than $100,000 annually, whether it is funded internally or externally, is required to have approval of the Board of Directors.

— Nancy Paris, Mercy Mobile Health Care, Atlanta, Georgia

The doing the job phase of your initiative is illustrative of the effort at large in that collaboration is essential to its success. This Core Process is non-linear. Your effort must maintain flexibility to keep pace with changing conditions in the community, and must creatively look on external forces as assets.

A few key considerations for the doing the job phase include the following:

- What is the role of our coalition in bringing about change and renewing our community?

- Where are the high-leverage change points?

- How do we manage the short term while we create the long term?

- How and when do we implement the necessary changes?

By the time your partnership has reached the doing the job stage there has been considerable inertia built up. Take advantage of this momentum and of the synergy that by now exists between Core Processes and use them to propel your initiative toward successful outcomes.

Potential Pitfalls and Strategies

Use the following worksheet as a way to brainstorm solutions for obstacles that might otherwise undermine your efforts.

Potential Pitfalls	Possible Strategies for Bypassing Pitfalls
1. "Turfism" creates an obstacle to forming new partnerships.	• Help smaller groups refocus from their own self-interest to that of the common good. • Remind stakeholders that by addressing the larger community issues, the general health and well-being will improve in the community, eventually yielding positive results for smaller groups as well. • Remember: there is strength in numbers.
2. Effort fails to recognize and therefore capitalize on all internal resources.	
3. Public communications and presentations seem to fall flat or generate little response.	
4. Funding instability arises.	
5. Effort's strength seems to be waning due to large expenditures of energy.	
6. Other Potential Pitfalls . . .	
7.	
8.	

ACTION WORKSHEET

Recruitment of Potential Partners

As your team prepares to do the job and steps back to consider all the potential partners in your community who might benefit from being involved in your initiative, use this worksheet to guide your efforts.

List potential partners (individual and organizational) and develop a strategy for contacting them:

Potential Partner	Information	Contacted When?	By Whom?

Monitoring and Adjusting

Develop shared ideas and values for a monitoring system

Clarify goals and objectives

Develop measures, tools and indicators

Develop evaluation design

Collect data

Synthesize and analyze data

Report results, findings and feedback

Recognize successes and challenges

Monitoring and Adjusting

Critical Success Factors

- Mutually agree on benchmarks and outcomes
- Build in monitoring mechanisms from the outset
- Use multiple methods to gather data
- Enable stakeholders themselves to monitor progress and identify roadblocks
- Continuously document, share and celebrate progress developments
- Use findings to immediately improve the effort

Coordinator and Staff	Coordinating Committee	Stakeholder One	Stakeholder Two	Stakeholder Three	Stakeholder Four
♫	**Step 1** — Develop shared ideas and values for a monitoring system • Is there consensus on what is to be publicly reported? • Have you reached consensus on values and expectations? ♫	♫	♫	♫	♫
♫	**Step 2** — Clarify goals and objectives ♫	♫	♫	♫	♫
Step 3 — Develop measures, tools and indicators ♫	♫				
♫	**Step 4** — Develop evaluation design • Does the steering committee approve the design? • Have you set priorities for monitoring and evaluation?				
♫	**Step 5** — Collect data • Do the data identify the problems? • Are the data collection methods clearly understood by all the participants? • Are the data relevant to shared vision values and expectations? ♫	♫	♫	♫	♫
♫	**Step 6** — Synthesize and analyze data ♫				
♫	**Step 7** — Report results, findings and feedback • Is there adequate feedback to stakeholders and beneficiaries? ♫				
♫	**Step 8** — Recognize successes and challenges ♫	♫	♫	♫	♫

♫ = Step is done by the corresponding partners as well as the initiator

This process was mapped by: Brenita Crawford, Steve Graham, Ted Landsmark, Jacquelyn Lendsey, William Powanda and Sarah Samuels

Monitoring and Adjusting

In this Core Process, all stakeholders play a role in measuring both the process and outcomes of the partnership. The information is gathered using a variety of tools and formats, and is done both formally and informally. Most important, the information gathered is used by stakeholders and the Committee to improve and sustain the partnership.

By evaluating your process and product as you go, your stakeholders will learn from accomplishments as well as mistakes. A good rule of thumb is to apply the learnings gained from your evaluations at the earliest juncture possible. This positive reinforcement will sustain the energy of the group and keep the effort from becoming mired in the difficulties presented by seemingly insurmountable obstacles.

Research as shown that implementing monitoring systems can yield both short- and long-term positive program effects. An example of a short-term effect of a safe sex campaign targeting teenagers would be increased awareness. The teens' understanding of the risks involved in engaging in unsafe sex may increase. Long-term, in direct correlation to meeting the short-term goals, this increased understanding may result in a decrease in sexually transmitted diseases in the educated population.

> By evaluating your process and product as you go, your stakeholders will learn from accomplishments as well as mistakes.

Monitoring and adjusting are ways of proactively evaluating your initiative's progress. Engaging in evaluation should help your group make decisions. Your partnership, therefore, should pick its priorities for monitoring and evaluation based on its questions and the areas in which decisions are likely to be needed.

▼

1. Develop shared ideas and values for a monitoring system.

Even in efforts with a great deal of trust and a shared vision, there can be significant differences in the way stakeholders view this Core

Process. It is therefore important to agree on the purpose and basic process for monitoring. Agreement should be reached by all stakeholders, as well as any Action Team charged with monitoring. Reaching agreement includes the following steps:

- Select evaluation methodologies appropriate to answering the main questions

- Decide on the balance between community ownership and process evaluation

- Agree on expectations regarding the level of evaluation

- Clarify who owns the data and interprets results

- Determine who will be involved in monitoring, and clarify their role

- Agree on how to handle community feedback

2. Clarify goals and objectives.

Once the overall purpose of monitoring has been agreed on, the partnership needs to determine exactly what it wishes to measure. There are a variety of ways to set targets for this achievement; you can use an absolute standard (100 percent or zero—the all-or-nothing approach), a normative standard (a benchmark based on what other comparable communities have achieved), or a relative standard (an improvement over current conditions in the community that can be feasibly obtained). Typically, an Action Team is charged with these steps:

- Determine benchmarks and outcomes before action begins (e.g., successful campaign to vaccinate 96 percent of preschool-age children may be considered a benchmark for success)

- Clarify how local health status indicators compare to state and national goals and data

- Gain consensus regarding what the most important data elements on indicators are

- Meet with key community leaders to gauge the effectiveness of preprogram communication versus actual program goals, objectives, etc.

- Evaluate staff progress in reaching program goals and objectives

- Assess program strengths and weaknesses

Having established one method of monitoring, Mercy Mobile Health Care moved on to clarify the goals and objectives for the second phase:

The Quality Improvement Task Force creates processes for monitoring client satisfaction. This year a method will be established to monitor collaborator or partnership satisfaction and involvement. Board members and volunteer surveys are also conducted annually.

— Nancy Paris, Mercy Mobile Health Care, Atlanta, Georgia

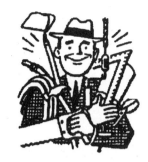

3. Develop measures, tools and indicators.

In this step, the Action Team determines how it will measure or monitor the partnership. The learnings from your community assessment may be useful here. Referring frequently to your shared vision and the community health indicators therein will also guide your efforts. Remain aware to

- Determine success targets for each initiative or action

- Create outcome and process objectives

- Distinguish between urgent, core and regular benchmarks

- Create mechanisms for capturing day-to-day, "ear to the ground" information about the partnership

- Identify outcomes data to collect from existing systems

- Determine early on which data are easily available

- Identify and develop new tools for measuring progress

- Involve all stakeholders in determining outcomes and benchmarks

> "Benchmarks will be organized and presented in ways that are understandable to the public."
>
> — Lynne Conner

Specific measurable indicators that represent the health status of Clark County will be produced and compared with standards (to be developed) that are consistent with the standards included in both the Washington State Public Health Improvement Plan and the National Health Promotion and Disease Prevention Objectives, Healthy People 2000. Benchmarks will be prepared to reflect each of the strategies that make up the Community Choices 2010 plan. They will be organized and presented in ways that are understandable to the public. Entitled "How Do We Measure Up?" the document includes three components: (1) indicators for the strategy areas with historical, current and goal information; (2) a summary outlining Community Choices 2010 and why community focus is important; and (3) an "issue" paper detailing sources, unavailable data, issues that were identified, and general committee comments.

— Lynne Conner, Community Choices 2010, Vancouver, Washington

4. Develop evaluation design.

Although developing your evaluation is something that your effort should be doing all along, this stage will formalize it. The design maps out how the measures and indicators will be linked and coordinated, who will gather the data, and other issues:

- Decide what data to collect, when to collect them, and who data will come from
- Review the linkage between initiatives and indicators
- Determine the frequency with which data will need to be updated
- Get technical assistance as needed

5. Collect data.

In this step, the partnership uses its measurement tools to collect data. This collection effort can include the following activities:

- Institute monitoring systems (e.g., periodically distribute questionnaires to the teenage population to monitor educational gains around a safe sex campaign)
- Implement a community survey to determine high-priority areas of interest and concern
- Send the survey out to community business organizations
- Develop and implement a database

 HCK2000 implements evaluation studies to monitor the progress being made toward the achievement of the HCK2000 objectives. HCK2000 partners with the Pacific Wellness Institute to implement an annual and sometimes semi-annual 5th, 6th or 7th grade survey to evaluate the progress and effectiveness of the Schools as Wellness Communities project. The grade level changes so we can follow the same students over a period of years. The data gathered are used in the Annual Report.

— Linda Zorn, Healthy Chico Kids 2000, Chico, California

6. Synthesize and analyze data.

This stage includes the following actions:

- Analyze and synthesize process and procedure data for the final report
- Use statistical measures as appropriate
- Frame findings in terms of public and community accountability
- Get technical assistance as needed

"The end result was a formal restructuring of the membership to include the broad-based representation of key stakeholders."

— Kathryn Wilson

7. Report results, findings, and feedback.

To ensure that the data are used to improve the partnership's performance, this step is critical. Data should also be user-friendly for a diverse audience and should reflect your effort's shared vision in its presentation. Considerations include the following:

- Combine process and outcome monitoring systems
- Provide feedback to all stakeholders
- Revise benchmarks yearly
- Measure evidence of initiative improvement based on evaluation findings

Partners for Prevention wanted to ensure their evaluation improved performance:

Partners did evaluate its strategic direction in 1994–95 through a process of retreats, informal focus groups and one-on-one interviews with key participants. The end result was a formal restructuring of the membership to include the broad-based representation of key stakeholders within the National City and Southeast San Diego communities. Participants who did not have a vested interest in the local communities were invited to participate as invited guests as opposed to voting partnership members.

— Kathryn Wilson, Partners for Prevention, National City, California

8. Recognize successes and challenges.

Partnerships can also use the findings as a basis for these actions:

- Organize topical forums or focus groups to share success stories as well as difficulties

- Document and analyze challenges so as to sidestep them in the future

- Celebrate successes

- Use media placements

According to Arthur T. Himmelman, "Commitments to ongoing assessment and evaluation in user-friendly formats provide community-based organizations with opportunities for monitoring the progress of the collaborative, both in its processes and products (outcomes)."

Abe Wandersman and Jean Ann Linney of the University of South Carolina advocate a four-step approach to assessment that may be useful:

1. Identify goals and desired outcomes

2. Assess the process (describe what you actually did, how much of it, and with whom)

3. Assess the outcomes (document what happened as a result of the program and which immediate or proximal changes occurred)

4. Assess the impact (examine the broader impact of the program on your community's well-being and the indicators of this)

The Action Worksheets in this section will elaborate on this four-step approach.

Be sure to conduct your evaluation within the context of action planning and doing the job so that the evaluation matches the goals of your effort. Consider the questions you want to have answered and have your data collection methods mirror them. Be sure that all evaluators provide information that meets the needs of the initiative, and implement the findings as soon as possible. Evaluation without adjustment is a hollow undertaking.

Potential Pitfalls and Strategies

Use the following worksheet as a way to brainstorm solutions for obstacles which might otherwise undermine your efforts.

Potential Pitfalls	Possible Strategies for Bypassing Pitfalls
1. Partners view continued action as more important than the evaluation of the effort.	• Consider that the partnership will more likely meet all stakeholders' needs if frequent evaluation and adjustment are built into the structure. • Remind stakeholders of an instance when quick evaluation saved precious time that would have been spent going in the wrong direction. • The old adage "a stitch in time saves nine" may serve to illustrate the value of monitoring and adjusting.
2. Hired evaluator dominates process without clear understanding of priorities.	
3. Evaluation methodology is distinct from effort's original goals.	
4. Stakeholders are unsure as to how to measure progress.	
5. Poor links to the community render feedback questionable.	
6. Other Potential Pitfalls. . .	
7.	
8.	

ACTION WORKSHEET

I. Identify Goals and Desired Outcomes

Part A: Make a list of the primary goals of the program

Ask yourself: "What were we trying to accomplish?" Check the goals that apply to your program and add any others on the lines provided.

✔	

Part B: Which groups did you *want* to involve?

Ask yourself: "Whom were we trying to reach?" Check the groups that apply to your program and add any others on the lines provided.

✔	Target Group	How many did you want to involve?

Part C: Which outcomes were desired?

Ask yourself: "As a result of this program, how would we like the participants to change? What would they learn? Which attitudes, feelings, or behavior would be different?" Check the outcomes that apply to your program and add any others on the lines provided.

✔	

Adapted from Linney, J.A., and Wandersman, A. (1991) *Prevention Plus III*. U.S. Department of Health and Human Services: Rockville, MD.

II. Process Assessment Worksheet

Program Type: _____

Part A: Which activities were planned?

Include a brief description of every program activity. Ask yourself: "What did we actually do to prepare for this and implement it?" Form a chronology of events constituting this program and a quantity indicator for each. For example, if one of the planned activities was the distribution of your vision statement to community members, indicate how many you had planned to distribute and how many were actually distributed.

Activity	Date	Quantity Planned	Quantity Actual

Quantity Totals

Number of activities _____ Length of time for each _____(hr)

Total hours of activity _____

List written materials available	How many available?	Total distributed

Other services delivered	Total

Adapted from Linney, J.A., and Wandersman, A. (1991) *Prevention Plus III*. U.S. Department of Health and Human Services: Rockville, MD.

Which topics or activities were planned but not covered?
What was the reason that these were not accomplished?

Activity	Reason for cancellation of activity

Part B: When was the program actually implemented (dates of activities, length of time for each), and who were the participants?

Date	Length of the activity	Percentage of time goal	Attendance	Percentage of attendance goal

Total number of activities	Total hrs	Percentage of goal	Total number (average of all sessions or activities)
_____	_____	_____	_____

Who was missing that you'd hoped to have participate in the program?

Which explanations can be offered for the discrepancy between the projected and the actual participation?

Part C: How did participants evaluate the activities?

Activity	Participants	Evaluation

Part D: What feedback can be used to improve the program for the future?

ACTION WORKSHEET

III. Outcome Assessment

The following evaluative device is designed to assist your efforts in determining and assessing your outcomes. Consider outcome to be predominantly short-term results. For example, in a teenage safe sex education program, the critical outcome measure would be improvement in safe sex practices among teenagers.

Program Type: _____

Desired Outcomes	Measure/Indicator	Observed Scores					Amount of Change	
		Project Group			Comparison Group		Before vs. after the project	Comparison group vs. project group
(list desired outcomes from Identifying Goals and Desired Outcome, part I.c)	(indicate the type of evidence you have for each outcome)	None	Before	After	Before	After		

Adapted from Linney, J.A., and Wandersman, A. (1991) *Prevention Plus III*. U.S. Department of Health and Human Services: Rockville, MD.

IV. Impact Assessment

Use this table to track the impact of your effort. Consider impact to be predominantly results (potentially long term) that affect health status. For example, in a teenage safe sex education program, reduction in HIV infection would demonstrate program impact.

Impact	Measure or Evidence	Project Group		Comparison Group		Amount of change
		Before	After	Before	After	

Adapted from Linney, J.A., and Wandersman, A. (1991) *Prevention Plus III*. U.S. Department of Health and Human Services: Rockville, MD.

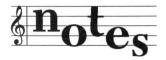

Four Case Studies

Community Collaboration in progress:

- **Growing Into Life**
  Aiken, South Carolina

- **Bethel New Life**
  Chicago, Illinois

- **Healthy Community 2000 of Mesa County**
  Grand Junction, Colorado

- **Healthy Communities Initiative of Greater Orlando**
  Orlando, Florida

Four Case Studies

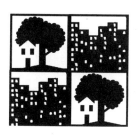

An Introduction

We derived the Core Processes in this book from focus groups, surveys, and work sessions with scores of people who have been working to transform their communities through partnership. We extracted from their widely varying experiences what seemed to be deep and constant, the stages and tasks through which every successful experience seems to pass.

To look at these processes in their natural environment, we did case studies of four communities. We intentionally picked four very different efforts—one in a dense inner-city district of Chicago, one in a rapidly growing Southern city, one in a small Southern town, and one in a rural Western county. Two were multicultural, one almost all African-American, one almost all white. Three set out on a planned course of community reconstruction, one grew organically over seventeen years.

Beneath all the differences, they had a lot in common—all of them set out to gather new energies to transform their communities. And all of them, in their own ways, used each of the Core Processes that we have discussed. The four case studies depict:

- Growing Into Life in Aiken, South Carolina
- Bethel New Life in the West Garfield Park district of Chicago
- Healthy Community 2000 initiative, the Civic Forum and the Community Health Assessment in Mesa County, Colorado
- Healthy Communities Initiative of Orlando, Florida

As you read each of these studies, compare each community to your own. Ask yourself what is the same and what is different. Ask yourself whether these techniques would work where you live, and how they might map onto your own efforts. Do you see, in these examples, assets that you could find at home, ways to do things that you have not tried, models for something that is missing from your work?

"Communities don't learn from statistics and studies," says Northwestern University's John McKnight. "They learn from stories."

Here are some stories.

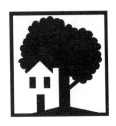

Aiken, Growing Into Life

Karen Papouchado nearly lost her job early on, and Steve Thompson, the city manager, has taken some hits due to the various controversies the effort spawned. But they do the right thing anyway. Things were falling apart and babies were dying in Aiken, South Carolina. And people wanted to do something.

Aiken is a charming Southern town of 20,000 not far from the Savannah River, on the Georgia border, a town of grand historic districts and lanes under arching live oaks. It had long been a winter place for the rich of New England, with soil that was considered "perfect for horses' hooves." The town is still peppered with Goodyears and Whitneys, and still is known for its polo grounds and equestrian paths.

Overlay that with nuclear physicists: in 1952 the U.S. Atomic Energy Commission, forerunner of the Department of Energy, opened the sprawling Savannah River Site nearby as a place to manufacture nuclear materials. It grew in time to become the state's single largest employer, with 26,000 workers spread over its 300 square miles. For nearly 40 years, it was the mainstay of the area's economy; the influx of Ph.D. scientists and engineers and their college-educated spouses from across the nation changed the culture. The town had always been warm—now it became sophisticated as well.

For most of those 40 years, the same mayor and city manager ran the quiet municipality. Things were tranquil and life was good.

But the turn of the 1990s brought a different kind of news. The Cold War ended, and suddenly the Savannah River site, now run by Westinghouse, started laying people off. By 1996 half its work force was gone, and many of the rest were employed not in nuclear weapons manufacture but in environmental restoration of the vast site, nearly pristine between the widely separated reactors, factories, and toxic waste dumps.

Several other things happened at about the same time. The state Department of Health and Environmental Control looked over the city's statistics and saw that Aiken County was among the worst in the state in infant mortality rates. And both the long-time mayor and the city manager retired. City governance was turned over to fresh new hands. "It was a shock when the local leadership changed" in the midst of so much turmoil, according to Barbara Strack, a local writer. "It was time to take measures to make sure that the town didn't get ruined. I don't know how many communities get that clarion a call."

Out of these disparate roots rose two separate efforts that coalesced in time to form a revolution for Aiken. As Karen Papouchado says, "The movement was truly organic and real."

In fact, we can start the story with Papouchado. In 1989, the state Department of Health and Environmental Control (DHEC) ranked the counties of South Carolina by their infant mortality rates. Aiken was the sixth worst, at 12.1 per 1,000 live births, far above the national average. DHEC put a grant together and looked for a local partner. They found that the local Mental Health Foundation, with Papouchado as chair, had widened its mandate to include the problem of children having babies. So they gave the foundation a grant with few instructions beyond "see what you can do about this problem."

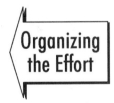

Assessing Current Realities and Trends

What Papouchado did was establish the Infant Mortality Task Force. The task force did three things right away. The first was to establish a Fetal and Infant Mortality Review (FIMR) board to review every baby's death. The second was a 12-page survey of 477 new mothers that turned up some sobering numbers. Nearly 60 percent of the new moms did not want their babies, 43 percent claimed to have been using birth control at the time of conception, 16 percent were under eighteen, 50 percent were on Medicaid, 33 percent had not had adequate prenatal care; 10 percent of the babies were underweight.

Organizing the Effort

The third assessment tool was the one that almost cost Papouchado her job. With the help of a professor at USC-Aiken, the task force sent a number of students into Aiken's public clinics asking for pregnancy information and testing. They wrote down the details of what happened to them—every indignity, delay, and unnecessary roadblock from the demoralized, underfunded staff—and Papouchado reported what she found.

The nurses and clinic managers were furious. Yet she was truly on the clinics' side. "People weren't getting the care they needed," says Papouchado (now mayor pro tem), "because the clinic staff was depressed, and felt it had no support from the community." The Health Department retrained the workers, and the task force organized a public-private partnership to refurbish the clinics.

Doing the Job

The task force's tactics for dealing with the appalling reality that they saw ranged from the classic, such as public information campaigns, better conditions at the clinics, and aggressive case management, to the innovative, such as prenatal ID cards and a 24-hour pregnancy line.

The city had already started a "community-oriented policing" (COPS) program, putting pairs of cops on bicycles in one high-crime community on a regular basis so that they could get to know people. COPS worked so well—drug use dropped 46 percent and violent crimes dropped 70 percent in that neighborhood in one year—that they expanded the program to another neighborhood and to the downtown area. They found apartments for several officers in the projects themselves, and other officers serve as substitute teachers in the public school system.

Then the task force recruited the officers for a critical task: identifying pregnant women and giving them a little information about the prenatal care that was available. For every 10 women referred, the officers got a free dinner at one of the town's better restaurants. The program was called "COPS and Moms."

Once you get policemen back in the community, even living in the projects, you increase the care and commitment level.

"Once you get policemen back in the community, even living in the projects," says Barbara Morgan, "you increase the care and commitment level." Morgan is the solicitor in Aiken, in effect the district attorney for a three-county area, and is now the chair of the task force. She came to realize that health was part of her job as she prosecuted more and more child abuse cases. She is hardly soft on crime: she has sent two murderers to the electric chair and another to a sentence of life without parole, in the past two years. Yet to her the involvement of law enforcement in the nurturing activities of the task force takes no great leap of imagination. "It's a natural progression. No one has to argue the causation here. Monsters do not spontaneously generate. You have to try to have an impact on the front end."

Monitoring and Adjusting

By 1993, when the rest of the strategic planning process was still gearing up, Aiken's infant mortality rate had dropped 40 percent to 7.2. The group's goal was 5.0, the level maintained by Japan.

But it was not enough. Infant mortality, though serious in itself, is but a red flag of deeper social problems. State statistics showed that Aiken County, with its 120,000 population, was the worst in the state in reports of child abuse and neglect, and in the proportion of children in foster care. The state as a whole was the worst in the country in infant mortality, and ranked 49th in SAT scores.

So by 1992 the task force had already expanded its original mission—to focus not only on infant mortality but also on domestic and child abuse, teen pregnancy, the lifestyle choices of young people, and poverty—and changed its name to "Growing Into Life."

The other half of the story began in 1992, with Steve Thompson, the new city manager. "He didn't have to convince anyone of the need to do something different," says Papouchado. "It was pretty clear."

Organizing the Effort

Rock Hill, South Carolina, had recently gone through a strategic planning process, and it had worked so well that the city manager had quit to start his own consulting firm. The City of Aiken organized a field trip, inviting 40 citizens from business, education, government, faith groups, media, and minority groups to travel the 100-mile width of the state to the North Carolina border for a two-day retreat to take a look at what Rock Hill had done. This Steering Committee liked what they saw so much that the City of Aiken hired Thompson, to the tune of some $40,000 over three years, to help them do the same. The city's budget for the entire process was more than $100,000.

Strategic planning, traditionally, is a simple process, involving just the top people in the organization, the finance department, and maybe a few consultants. This would be different. Called "Planning Today For Tomorrow," the three-year effort would involve more than 300 citizens on 12 committees doing six-month studies of such areas as economic development, education, community building, senior life, safety, the environment, and culture. Growing Into Life became the health arm of the planning effort.

Convening the Community

"It comes down to your old-fashioned networking," according to Strack. As Papouchado puts it: "This stuff comes right out of kindergarten—you've got to like these people, you've got to be friends with them. You don't have to like everybody, but have to have enough friends that other people don't want to be left out. You establish personal relationships, you work by obligations. People who know how to make things work will know what I'm talking

It comes down to your old-fashioned networking.

about. You work through the 200 or 300 people you know, no matter how big the town is. You do that, and it's not that hard to get these things accomplished."

But networking by itself was not enough. In the end, only about one-third of the group was invited by city officials. The other two-thirds called in response to ads that the city put in the paper explaining the project and asking for volunteers.

"A lot of diversity came from those ads," says Strack. The African-American community showed up in droves, and the Hispanic community turned out to be larger than anyone suspected. It had grown rapidly since the last census, and was well dispersed throughout the community. The newly arrived Hispanics thought of Aiken as "heaven on earth," says Strack—friendly, safe, and free of discrimination.

In the end, everyone was involved—African-American, Hispanic, white, school kids, homemakers, entrepreneurs, seniors, city officials. The group even consulted a prisoner for his ideas on crime prevention.

Once the 25-member committees were filled, scores of other people demanded to know why they had not been included—and they soon were put to work.

A town document describes the liveliness of the ensuing process:

Organizing the Effort

> The groups developed very individual leadership styles. Some met before 7 A.M. every week; some needed food and drink to keep them going in the afternoons; and others scurried from work and soccer practice to make evening meetings. The groups devoured information and made site visits all over the city and into nearby states. Requests to travel to other countries were cheerfully denied by the city manager. Controversy erupted in almost every group. Members stated that they would walk out if certain subjects were to be considered, and they did, only to come back because they couldn't stand not knowing what was being hatched in their absence. Each committee had co-chairpersons, and the chairs of the Families group nearly came to blows over a basic difference in leadership styles.

While most community partnership efforts work out their shared vision as a whole, in Aiken it was in the individual groups where people did most of the work toward a shared vision. It was the first item on the agenda. This, too, was lively. As the town document puts it:

Creating a Shared Vision

> This aired most of the controversies immediately. What was good health care? Who got it and who didn't? Why couldn't it be like it used to be when Dr. Jones made house calls? Who wants academic tracking? What about cooperative learning? We want neighborhood schools! We don't need industry—just send everyone who's moved here in the past 5 years away! I won't let you talk about recreation until you give me more facilities in the minority section.

In the end, each committee came up with a shared vision. For the battling Families group, it took a visit by Papouchado and one of the co-chairs to a national meeting at Jimmy Carter's Interfaith Health Studies Center in Atlanta before they could all see eye-to-eye on the role of religion in Aiken's future. But eventually they, too, found consensus.

After many months of work, the Planning Today For Tomorrow task force brought forward scores of separate, specific goals—such as "cut teen pregnancy by 50 percent," "construct a Visitors Reception Center," and "build a back entrance to the airport"—grouped in four general categories:

Action Planning

- "The Family City," including healthcare, retirement, community services, culture and the arts

- "The Business City," including education and economic development

- "The Green City," including recreation and tourism, and the city's growth strategy

- "The Historic City," including residential infill (enticing more new and refurbished housing into neighborhoods close to the center of town, instead of the edges), and preserving and enhancing the historic downtown

Each group of goals listed specific actions, along with which organization or partnership took responsibility for that action (such as "City and county: renovate Farmers' Market" or "Aiken Corporation: Construct spec building for Ventures Industrial Park"). The actions and responsibilities were specific enough, and set out clearly enough, that they could be tracked.

People say: you're doing entirely too many things, you can't sustain it, but it's sustaining itself, and it's breeding as it goes.

In planning actions, says Papouchado, "We tapped into what each group could bring to the table—the health department is doing this, the hospital is doing that, let's put them together. It was really simple. Everybody had the energy to do something."

The final plan was approved at the opening of a permanent display center downtown, complete with models, video-enhanced drawings, and plans.

Doing the Job

To the delight and astonishment of many locals, the action plans are being accomplished. "People come in with their checklists, saying, 'This one's done, we're a few months late on this other one.'"

No sooner had the plans been made final than the fundraising cranked up. The city, the Chamber of Commerce, and the Downtown Development Corporation started Aiken 20/20, pledging to raise $3.5 million in 1994 to start carrying out the plan. By the time the plan entered its public phase in October 1994, private sources had already pledged more than $1.5 million.

"People say: you're doing entirely too many things, you can't sustain it," says Papouchado. "But it's sustaining itself, and it's breeding as it goes."

Monitoring and Adjusting

"At times we have had to change our focus," says Strack, "sometimes quickly. We had been focused on domestic violence. Then the state passed a draconian welfare reform law—two years and you're out, the mother has a job or you're off the rolls—and suddenly we need to find child care for 800 children, and we have to make sure that kids are not starving on the streets."

Other parts of the project involved a lot of back-and-fill, trial and error, and learning as they went. For instance: "We missed an incredible number of people the first time through," says Papouchado, "especially blue-collar people in the housing projects. We connected with them over the last year and a half through our 'Stone Soup' project, which uses John McKnight–style 'asset mapping.' We targeted four neighborhoods, sought out and convened people we identified as emerging leaders, trained them, worked with them, and sent them back into the neighborhoods. It really worked. We've adopted into the strategic plan."

Convening the Community

Two key people had refused to get involved: the town's African-American obstetricians. They were not hostile to the project or its goals; they just felt that they were far too busy to attend all those meetings. Yet if there was no way to involve them in planning, still there was a way to reach them by action. Growing Into Life simply asked them whether they would like to have a little help: a county nurse working in each of their offices. Their surprised answer was, "Of course." Growing Into Life has had to do without their insight, but it is now working closely with them.

Here and elsewhere, Healthier Communities efforts often serve as seedbeds for other projects. As a spin-off of the Aiken effort, local Hispanics became far more aware of themselves and their needs and capacities. As a first effort, they organized to teach their children English before they reached school age.

Not that it's all been easy. "Whenever local government is going to be involved, you encounter hornets' nests," says Papouchado who is mayor pro tem. "We had fire storms more intense than I ever could have imagined. Public art can really sink your ship, for instance. To illustrate the point of creating visual accents scaled for a civic axis, the person doing the computer renditions replaced the little fountain downtown with a big horse statue on a pylon. We were inundated with calls, saying, "Don't move the fountain!" We set to build more bike paths. If anything could be innocuous and safe to be in favor of, you would think it would be a bike path. But we got a lot of people that are one step beyond the NIMBYs, the 'Not In My Back Yard' folks. I call these people BANANAs—'Build Absolutely Nothing Anywhere Near Anything.' Every neighborhood had objections. They feared crime, of all things. But we persevered, and now we are building our bike path.

"Another part of our plan involved annexation: The city has grown around some 'doughnut holes' of unincorporated land. This creates problems for public safety and city services. We got on the wrong side of a local senator, and he was able to block our annexation efforts at the state level. So we just got around it with our terms of service agreements. If any property in those enclaves changes hands, they will have to renew their contracts for public services from the city—and we won't renew unless they join the city. Our unofficial motto is: 'Over, Under, Around, and Through.' If we can't do it one way, we'll do it another."

This flexibility seems key to the whole effort, even when it comes to planning. "We try to have a plan," says Papouchado, "But if some-

If we can't do it one way, we'll do it another.

one has energy for something that is a little different from our plan, we'll regroup around that." For instance, one project for bringing Aiken together arose after the planning effort, and is already at work. Two 20-something computer entrepreneurs recently just plopped into town and decided to adopt it. In collaboration with the City of Aiken, they started a local Intranet featuring information about the town for residents and tourists alike, and promised to staff it 24 hours a day, making Aiken one of only half a dozen such "wired" towns in the nation (http://www.aiken.net).

Monitoring and Adjusting

The task force has quarterly meetings, and out of the meetings the city publishes publish quarterly reports with updates on all the projects.

Monitoring progress is often a continuation and refinement of the original assessment process. In 1996, in fact, Aiken secured a large grant from the March of Dimes to do a baseline survey of 50 measures, from air quality to the school dropout rate. And the state has asked the original FIMR board to expand its purview to include all deaths of people under 18 years of age in the county.

One task force document summarized three important factors that worked in Aiken's favor: leadership, collaboration, and financing:

> Leadership in Aiken is well defined, with established leaders who are respected and with up-and-coming leaders who are supported because the community knows that sustained change occurs only with leadership that will carry the vision forward. Time-consuming ventures like strategic planning still attract busy leaders because support systems are in place to keep meetings organized, to handle paperwork, and to manage the flow of the project.

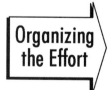

Organizing the Effort

> The second factor influencing success is collaboration. The task force modeled this by creating itself outside of any existing agency or government structure. Led by high-profile health champions and supported by dedicated "worker bees," the task force eschewed red tape and solved problems by talking to each other. Small successes led to bigger ones, until now the task force is the "grease" in bureaucratic gears. The same paradigm transferred to the Strategic Plan where cooperation showed itself to be non-threatening and even exhilarating.

> The third factor is financing. Without funding, plans sit on shelves. The City of Aiken budgeted well for three years of

planning, and the other business and industry members contributed generously to implement the vision. Aggressive grant-seeking, partnerships among providers, and in-kind services have added to the resources. When everyone is included from the beginning, everyone seems to have something to offer.

"Stop" really isn't in the vocabulary here.

The whole process so far has gone with surprising smoothness. "There have been almost no power struggles," says Strack. "People wind up on opposite sides of various issues, they run against each other for office, but still they know that Growing Into Life and the planning effort are too important to risk."

"Turf issues?" asks Papouchado. "All you have to do is roll over. You can't have a dog fight if one of the dogs rolls over. That's one reason that Growing Into Life is not even incorporated as a 501c3. We can't take the money that would go to another group—we don't even exist."

"The problem is beyond anyone's turf, so the solution has to be," says Morgan. "If you're not going at it to win for someone or to make someone lose, you can forget the 'mud-puddle issues' and get on the solution road. Once you get the taste that you can do something, it gets easy."

"In the early years," says Strack, "the task force moved mountains that they thought could not be moved. 'Stop' really isn't in the vocabulary here. People give up and go away, or they come to a consensus. You've got to get along because you will be here for generations—even those who moved recently just start to take that attitude on. It's almost a rebirth experience—let's see if we can reinvent ourselves. We won't get another chance."

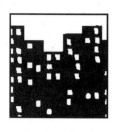

Chicago, Bethel New Life

It was a violent, scary, rundown, hopeless place. Then Mary Nelson came to stay. After thirty years, it's still violent, still scary, and now it's drug-ridden. But parts of it are not so rundown. And none of it is as hopeless as it was.

Nelson didn't mean to stay. She just meant to help her brother move. He was a Lutheran minister, with a new assignment: the Bethel Lutheran Church in a neighborhood called West Garfield Park in Chicago. A map shows Garfield Park to be an expanse of greenery with two lakes and a grand botanical conservatory about four miles straight west from the Loop on the Eisenhower Expressway or the Lake/Dan Ryan El (the "Green Line"). Just beyond it, the 107 blocks of West Garfield Park can look deceptively genteel with their arches of trees. The numbers reveal some of what's beneath that leafy surface: 45 percent of the population on public assistance—more than half of them for four years or more. Nearly 30 percent of the births are to teenage mothers, and 64 percent of the households are led by single parents, so perhaps it is not surprising that nearly 60 percent of the children live in poverty. Two-thirds of all high school students drop out, and 62 percent of adults have no high school diploma. In both 1992 and 1993, the police district that includes West Garfield Park counted 94 murders, the highest in all Chicago.

When David Nelson and his 25-year-old sister Mary arrived in 1965, the locals were throwing bricks at the National Guard and turning over police cars. The Nelsons had every reason to fear for their lives. After all, they were not only new to the area, they were white, like the police, the National Guard, and everyone in authority, almost without exception. The people throwing the bricks were African-American.

David and Mary Nelson decided to try again another day. But when they came back two days later the bricks were still flying. In fact, their car got hit with bricks as they came off the expressway. The heck with it, they decided, they might as well stay.

Mary felt she couldn't just help her brother unpack and then run off and leave him in such a volatile situation. She would stay until the tensions eased. They didn't ease. There were five riots in the neighborhood over the next four years. By then Mary Nelson was deeply involved in the community.

It ran in the family. David and Mary's father was a Lutheran minister in Washington, D.C. Her other brother was also a Lutheran minister. Her sister had married one. The guest room in their childhood home had always been full of strangers down on their luck or just out of prison. Her parents had spent a lot of their time working with the poor of Washington. It came with the territory. After getting a master's degree in urban education from Brown University, Mary had gone off to build schools and teach in Tanzania for two years. Now, in West Garfield Park, she became a part of her brother's ministry, helping with "social action" such as starting an alternative high school for dropouts and 17 daycare centers.

The $9,600 has become a $10 million annual budget.

Bethel was part of a consortium of Westside Chicago churches called Westside Isaiah, named after a striking passage in the prophetic book:

> If you put an end to oppression, to every gesture of contempt, and to every evil word; if you give food to the hungry and satisfy those who are in need, then the darkness around you will turn to the brightness of noon. And I will always guide you and satisfy you with good things. I will keep you strong and well. You will be like a garden that has plenty of water, like a spring of water that never goes dry. Your people will rebuild what has long been in ruins, building again on the old foundations. You will be known as the people who rebuilt the walls, who restored the ruined houses. (Isaiah 58: 9–12)

In 1979 the Nelsons and the people of Bethel Lutheran decided to take the passage literally. After all, it was pretty clear, especially the part about restoring the "ruined houses." There were plenty of ruined houses in West Garfield Park. The housing stock was rapidly deteriorating. Some 200 units a year were boarded up and abandoned, decent places to live were scarce, and home ownership was increasingly out of reach of the residents. Somebody should rebuild the houses, and help the residents buy them. Who better than the church?

But the other Westside churches would have none of it. The housing business was too capital-intensive, they said, and it was far beyond their expertise. So Bethel did it alone. They passed the hat among themselves. David and Mary borrowed on their credit cards. All together they came up with $9,600.

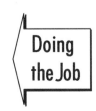

Doing the Job

For $275, HUD gave them an old three-flat apartment building it had foreclosed, and the people of Bethel Lutheran rehabilitated it.

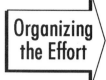

The effort grew from that thin beginning. They incorporated as Bethel New Life. Five times they put the church in hock to try the next project. But they did more than survive. Bethel has, at this point, built or rehabilitated more than 1,000 units of housing and sold them to residents by underwriting no-down-payment "sweat equity" deals. The $9,600 has become a $10 million annual budget.

And the mission has expanded. It became obvious very early that no level of housing is affordable to people who don't have jobs. The official level of unemployment among adults in West Garfield Park was 27 percent, the true level far higher. So Bethel started an Employment and Training Services initiative that has placed more than 4,000 people in full employment.

In attempting to place people in full employment, Bethel ran up against another stark reality: People can't work if they are not healthy, or if they have to stay home to take care of a family member who is ill. So the organization developed, over time, a variety of healthcare services for children, teens, working-age people, and seniors.

In the mid-1990s, Bethel itself employs some 450 people, and the array of programs that Bethel has developed to meet specific needs is impressively broad. It includes

Housing

- 1,000 units of housing
- Some 30 loan packages put together and brokered each year
- The Westside Isaiah Plan (20 Westside churches committed to building 250 new homes)

Jobs and training

- An employment center that places an average of more than 500 people a year in full-time jobs, and works with other agencies to provide literacy and training programs
- Several businesses owned and run by young people, including a bookstore, a credit union, and a catering business, all based in the local high school
- A summer youth program hiring young people for projects such as voter registration and crime watches

- Training programs to help welfare mothers enter the work force, including one that turns them into licensed daycare operators and helps them buy and rehabilitate their homes

Economic redevelopment

- Beth-Anne Life Center, the 9.2-acre campus of the former 437-bed St. Anne's hospital, which Bethel has bought and is turning into housing, offices, a retail shopping complex, a small business "incubator," a training center for daycare operators, a performing arts center, a large regional primary healthcare center, and (in partnership with IBM) a Training Institute providing computer training, literacy, and pre-employment skills in a modern office setting

- "Targeted Neighborhoods" in four neighborhoods (so far), each encompassing four to twelve square blocks: convening the community, helping create a new vision for the area, and providing the help that the neighborhood needs to begin to realize the vision

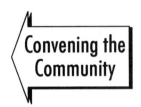

Convening the Community

- A technology-transfer partnership with Argonne National Laboratory, creating new businesses in industrial site environmental assessment, housing energy efficiency, and recycling services (including a $1.4 million Materials Recovery Facility), as well as providing young people with training and career opportunities in urban and environmental engineering

- Participation in developing the Northwest Industrial Corridor (bordering West Garfield Park on the north) as one of the city's Model Industrial Corridors

- A $3 million city rehab of the local public library (sparked by Bethel) and building two self-help parks

Health

- Bethel Holistic Health Center, which provides family health services, through three FTE physicians and a nurse practitioner, to more than 1,000 residents a month

- The Community Wellness Initiative, a joint effort with the Westside Health Authority

- A lead abatement program

- Healthy Moms, Healthy Kids, which provides case management and tracking to more than 2,000 families

- Health fairs

- AIDS counseling and education

- A campaign to reduce infant mortality that cut the rate from 33 per 1,000 in the mid-1980s to 21 per 1,000

Seniors

- Subsidized housing for seniors

- Senior home repair

- Adult daycare, meals, and home care services for seniors

Social action

- A *Take Back the Streets* campaign, in which local residents and church groups create street fairs, teach African dancing, start basketball tournaments, hold prayer vigils, and sell sno-cones and hot dogs on the corners to create street life and compete with the drug sellers for sidewalk "turf," while offering them Bethel's jobs and training programs. Planning for this collaborative effort involved the city, the alderman's office, churches, schools, block clubs, business organizations, and the police. The initial 40-day intensive effort focused on a six-block area that had the worst drug-dealing problem. The city helped by demolishing abandoned buildings and sending prisoners to clean up vacant lots. Others collaborated in such actions as installing more security devices and lighting, hiring more security guards, and putting fences around vacant lots.

- A vigorous protest movement launched when the city said it planned to shut down the "Green Line" elevated train, which runs through West Garfield Park. The line stayed—and the local Lake/Pulaski station became the center of a $300 million city redevelopment effort anchored in one of Bethel's "Targeted Neighborhood" initiatives. New investment included a major shopping center, a branch bank, a police substation, and a daycare center. Bethel, other members of the coalition that stopped the shutdown, the Neighborhood Capital Budget Group, the Center for Neighborhood Technology, and an architectural firm collaborated on the plans.

- A "re-neighboring" program in which people get to know the people who live close to them.

- A campaign to foster the cleanliness and safety of neighborhoods through "clean up, green up" days, block clubs, youth employment, and police substations.

- Family support services for mothers and children who are homeless or on public assistance, including transitional housing for some 20 families a year.

- A volunteering program led by a staff volunteer coordinator.

In 1994, in response to a federal program creating "Empowerment Zones," Bethel New Life led the creation of the West Garfield Park Empowerment Zones Collaborative. This collaborative brought together a number of coalitions and partnerships that had formed over the years, with Bethel taking the lead in many of them. Thirteen organizations committed as "core" groups and seventeen others participated in the planning and visioning, and gave assistance in one form or another.

Convening the Community

The Collaborative started with a series of open community meetings that mixed invited "experts" and stakeholders with anyone who wanted to come. The purpose of these meetings was simply to gather information about what different organizations were doing or planning in the community.

Assessing Current Realities and Trends

The next series of meetings, held at the "Gold Dome" in Garfield Park, had a different purpose: creating a holistic vision of a healthy, sustainable community. Thirty to forty people showed up for each session.

Creating a Shared Vision

A "writing committee" took the results of the "Gold Dome" meetings and expressed that vision in a series of initiatives, most of them building on efforts that Bethel had started. They sent the results to anyone who wanted to see them, asking for input, making changes as a consensus emerged. As described in a Bethel document, the ten resulting initiatives are

Action Planning

- Expansion and enhancement of an industrial corridor to bring in new industry and liveable-wage jobs, focused on environmental or recycling-related manufacturing companies

- Commercial development around an existing elevated train stop . . . in concert with extensive renovations undertaken by the city

- Construction of a Family Wellness Center that brings existing community-based family services and state programs together in a coordinated, integrated delivery system

- Housing redevelopment in four focused areas, creating a critical mass with security and a rewoven sense of neighborhood

- A campaign to create neighborhood safety and cleanliness through police substations, youth employment, block clubs, clean green-up days, and reduction of liquor stores

- Enhancement of the Garfield Park Conservatory, creating a tourist attraction, training ground, and opportunity for related commercial development

- Employment and training in partnership with the Argonne National Laboratory, focused on the environmental field, with a related urban engineering track for high school students

- Creation of a network of community-based health centers enabling accessible, quality health care with a focus on outreach, preventions and self-help

- Expansion of the Youth Enterprise Network, a vocational education reform initiative wherein high school students set up their own businesses linked to community economic development

- Expansion and enhancement of the community's existing commercial strip

A different model

Bethel New Life is quite different from the other efforts that we have featured here. It has been described as a "grassroots" effort, as opposed to "top-down" efforts like those in Orlando and Aiken, which start with the most powerful local people (mayor, newspaper publisher, city manager) and proceed outward and downward. The differences are instructive:

1. Organic structure—The "top-down" model involves gathering a sense of the entire community into an overarching vision, and proceeding from that vision into specific projects. Bethel New Life began as one specific project—affordable housing— and grew organically to take up other challenges, such as jobs, health, senior services, and economic development, as a series of specific, expanded answers to the knot of questions presented by this enormously challenged community.

2. Overt basis in Christian faith—Other efforts involve religion at one level or another. One of the roots of the Orlando effort was clearly the passionate belief in doing the right thing for the community, a belief held by most of the people who run Florida Hospital, an Adventist institution, as well as by many of the others who were involved. But Bethel New Life, though organizationally separate from Bethel Lutheran and the churches of Westside Isaiah, carries its Christian message and motivation much closer to the surface. When the "Take Back the Streets" campaigners tell the young drug runners that "there is another way," they don't just mean job training programs and entrepreneurial training. In this context, they clearly also mean "The Way," a life based in the church, personal responsibility, and commitment to family.

3. Slow evolution over time—The "top-down" model starts all at once. It seemingly has to, since it is necessary for the community as a whole to grasp a new gestalt of itself and to proceed from this new vision to new actions. Bethel New Life evolved bit by bit.

Which is correct?

Which is the right model? Is the "top-down" model, developed under the rubric of "Healthy Cities" or "Healthy Communities" by Len Duhl and Trevor Hancock, the World Health Organization, the National Civic League and The Healthcare Forum—the "gather everyone and create a vision" model—better? Or is the Bethel New Life "grow organically through faith and trial" model better?

The evidence at hand suggests that neither is right—in the sense that neither is a magic wand that transforms communities overnight—and that both are right, that both models can have enormous transformative power. Furthermore, the study of change in chaotic systems suggests that any transformation that works over the long haul must arise organically out of specific local circumstances—every change that works will happen differently.

Seventeen years into the attempt, Bethel New Life seems to be succeeding wonderfully. A more fruitful question than whether it is using the correct model might be: What are the specific local circumstances that allow this model to work so well?

You can do it. If you don't do it, who will?

More than any of the other communities we have studied, West Garfield Park is a homogeneous community, almost a monoculture, an urban African-American culture undergirded by Protestant Christian churches. By and large, proposing a specifically Christian vision of community renewal is not divisive, but unifying. It calls people back to their roots and their family.

On the other hand, West Garfield Park is at war with itself. The community is still trying to answer the basic question of how to survive, at the very bottom of Maslow's hierarchy of needs, and in West Garfield Park there are two starkly different, competing answers to that question. One is crime, especially drug dealing. The other is getting a job, getting an education, taking personal responsibility, and making a commitment to family. This divided consciousness is not helped by the fragmented and too often corrupt, ethnic-based political leadership of Chicago. An attempt to gather a consensus in all of West Garfield—or in all of Chicago—might awaken many competing demons, and ultimately fail. It might be more fruitful in such circumstances to start with one small project, sink deep roots, and grow slowly.

West Garfield Park is a place of scarce resources. In Bethel New Life, this is coupled with a ferocious focus on being homegrown. In John McKnight's terms, the effort arises out of the "gifts and capacities" of the community itself, and the control, management, and benefits of the effort stay in the community. Bethel is not at all bashful about using government money, or assistance from foundations and corporations—in fact, a great deal of its effort could be described as various ways of seeking out, managing, and leveraging that help. But to have the ability to attract and use these outside resources without being controlled from the outside, Bethel had to grow the infrastructure—the staff, the expertise, the track record. It is questionable whether it could have done any of that quickly.

Finally, West Garfield Park has strong local leadership, apparently dedicated to the community, patient, indefatigable, skillful, whose rewards seem to come from the work itself, not from any results of the work. Mildred Wiley, Bethel's director of community organizing, says of this need for very special leadership: "You can do it. If you don't do it, who will?" We each have the necessary leadership in ourselves, she says, "because you recognize that there's something wrong." If such leadership had not come forward in the community, the only hope for renewal would come from the outside, from the "top down."

Bethel's method seems to fit the ground from which it grew. Could it have grown faster if it had employed what was later developed as the "Healthy Cities/Healthy Communities" model? We have no way of knowing. This is not a laboratory experiment. We have no parallel universe in which we can try it the other way. But it is possible. It is also possible that such an effort, with shallower roots and a more rapidly built infrastructure, may have run into serious problems, or simply died off, without reaching the longevity and success that this effort has. This certainly was the fate of many grandiose efforts of the sixties and seventies.

Now that it is well established, Bethel is using the "top-down" model in certain targeted neighborhoods. These "Focused Area Development" initiatives begin at the very beginning, with volunteers going door-to-door; asking people what they think the opportunities, assets, and needs of the neighborhood are; and asking whether people were willing to come to a meeting. Bethel has at least one part-time staff member attached to the project living in the targeted area. Bethel convenes the community, seeks input, helps them shape it into a vision, brings in architects to render that vision into architectural sketches and renderings, then provides the neighborhood with the help, access to capital, and experience it needs to make the changes.

To students of community development, Bethel's methods seem sharply reminiscent of the "asset-based" development ideas advocated by John McKnight and John Kretzmann of Northwestern University. This is no coincidence: It was in studying Bethel (among other places) that they developed many of those ideas. "Academics have to come with a kind of humility," says Nelson, "knowing that the answers come out of an honest-to-goodness collaborative process. The ideas have to come out of the people who struggle with it every day. Your study won't be any good unless it's action research, where you're in process all the time. Too often people in academic settings have a mindset that says, 'We studied all these years, so we have these answers.' The mindset blocks hearing what people in non-academic settings have to say. The reason our collaboration with Argonne National Laboratories works so well is that they have a genuine feeling that we are in this together, that they don't have all the answers. For them, the work is a process of scientific discovery, and the answers could come out of either one of us. It's the quality of the leadership there, they are looking for that 'Aha!' feeling. When they call themselves our 'partners,' they really mean it."

> The reason our collaboration with Argonne National Laboratories works so well is that they have a genuine feeling that we are in this together, that they don't have all the answers.

All elements present

Despite the different shape of the model, all the elements that we have presented as part of our model show up in Bethel's model also, though sometimes in a form that better fits the local circumstances.

Convening the Community

Though Bethel New Life did not grow out of any grand convention of all West Garfield Park, there is no question that it continually takes the temperature of the neighborhoods. Besides the specific convening of targeted neighborhoods, Bethel regularly does formal surveys about specific questions. And situated as it is, arising out of the local churches, with all of its 400 staff members living in the community, there is little separation between what "the public" wants and what Bethel hears. In this respect, it is of great importance that few of the staff have much, if any, training in such things as large-scale real estate rehabilitation, equity financing, and economic development—and that they see their inexperience as an asset. They are forced to turn outward, to seek the opinions of the neighborhood and the guidance of their Advisory Board members.

Creating a Shared Vision

Similarly, Bethel New Life has never attempted to help all of West Garfield Park articulate a shared vision expressed in concrete goals. Yet the shared vision is there, precisely because it is not a heterogeneous, fractionated culture, but a single culture split between two ways of surviving. Those who are advocating the path represented by Bethel already have a shared vision, articulated in the passage from Isaiah. They have developed the concrete expressions of that vision as they have moved forward: first, affordable housing, then decent jobs, then health, and on to community development, neighborhood revitalization, and safe streets.

In its "Focused Area Developments" and specific projects, Bethel goes to great extremes to create a truly shared vision. "In one area, for instance," says Nelson, "we started with the public school, American National Bank, and a local church. We went through eight neighborhood meetings to identify the assets of the area. The vision that came out of that process included traffic calming circles, play spaces for the kids, and a lot of other things. We got the park district involved. The local school council was very suspicious for the first few meetings. Trying to get them bought in took some private meetings."

The information that Bethel needs in order to decide what the community needs is not scarce. It is all around them—almost all of the staff live in the community. Usually there is little necessity to do further research to establish a need for a specific program. More often it is a question of doing something about a problem that is glaringly obvious and has been for years. "Because we are church-based," says Nelson, "every Sunday morning people are pulling on your sleeve to say 'Hey, we have to do this.' You have to do this in a neighborly way, instead of saying that you have all the answers. This neighborhood is a live being, it takes all of us to make it work. Folks in the neighborhood may not say things the right way. When you start really interacting with people who are living with it every day, the first thing you're going to get is a lot of negativism. You have to be tough enough to live through that, then pose some possibilities and opportunities. I'm action-oriented, I don't pause enough to listen. It's when you start hearing things coming through in different words that you know people are really interested in it. They're telling you, 'We gotta do something about this.'"

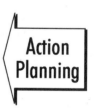

Assessing Current Realities and Trends

In addition to this constant informal conversation, Bethel does gather an enormous amount of data. It combines the data that are available from government and other sources with its own surveys, door-to-door "outreach," and data from its wellness programs, with participation in block clubs, community forums, business organizations, and churches.

One of the advantages of a slow evolution is that it involves a lot of trial-and-error, which is a slower but surer method of communal learning. "In collective planning," says Nelson, "you have to have someone who virtually stays on the telephone making sure that all the key actors are kept informed—the principal of the school, the police liaison, the alderman's office—coaxing, letting people know that people feel their ideas are important, getting back to everyone, typing up the notes from the meeting, sending them out to everyone that came. That intense organizing function is messy, but it's the key to success, for us."

Action Planning

Wiley points out that, once you get people involved in a project, "You've got to have something that you can finish, something visually different, whether it's a building demolished, or a more visible police presence, within six months to a year, or you'll lose them."

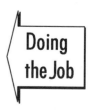

Doing the Job

The projects planned by Bethel have certain qualities in common besides being good for the community. They often have some immediate, visible benefit. They actually employ people from the community.

And they have a "multiplier effect": They produce goods and services that go on to draw more money and stability into the community.

That intense organizing function is messy, but it's the key to success, for us.

One example is the daycare program. Bethel's staff observed two linked problems: Many women could not take a job because they had young children or aged parents at home, and there was no affordable daycare—and many women had no training or licensing necessary for a job. The solution? Train some women to be daycare providers and help them get their licenses, turning the skills they had into something marketable. Help them upgrade their homes (and in several dozen cases, help them buy the home) to be licensed as small daycare centers. The result: entrepreneurial opportunities, income and home ownership for some women, affordable daycare and the opportunity to work for many others.

Monitoring and Adjusting

Because they are specific, targeted efforts, most of Bethel's initiatives require no special monitoring or re-surveys. It is easy to keep track of the number of people moved into permanent jobs, the number of new homeowners, a drop in infant mortality. Still, Bethel staff articulates explicit goals for most initiatives. The Argonne partnership, for instance, will be measured primarily by the number of jobs it produces. Other measurements will include the number of young people who successfully navigate the training-internship program through college to a career in engineering; the number of housing units renovated using the Argonne technology; and the number of area residents trained in site assessment and remediation.

The success of other efforts, such as the "Take Back the Streets" campaign, is not so easy to track, and there is no clear method for monitoring progress.

Report back your successes to people who have given money, effort, or political support, to be able to say, "See? It made a difference."

Is this a problem? Could be. But there are reasons to believe that it is not that much of a problem. We monitor progress for two reasons: One is to check how we are doing. Do we need mid-course corrections? The other reason is to be able to report back your successes to people who have given money, effort, or political support, to be able to say, "See? It made a difference."

If you are doing something like cleaning up a river, you will need some numbers and scientific tests to monitor your progress—so many parts per million of this pollutant, so many of that one. If you are cleaning up a street corner, such numbers are a lot harder to come by. Is it more effective to set up an ice cream stand on the corner, or to have choir practice there? Are any of the young men coming in for job training actually drug runners? Yet numbers may be less relevant than educated personal observations. A street that is a drug haven is not hard to spot—no families hanging out on the street, just young males, even on a hot summer evening; the young men not playing basketball or talking loudly, just hanging; cars cruising slowly; whispered conversations; guys draped over the public phone, as if waiting for it to ring. When the organization, like Bethel, has a tight, intermeshed relationship with the community it is trying to transform, simply noticing the effect of their actions is often sufficient feedback for mid-course corrections.

The primary reason that we need to report back successes in most community initiatives is that the people who are working together have little experience with each other. An organization that has grown up organically, building a long track record with the community, with sponsors and advisors, has built a level of trust that makes it less necessary to report successes on each initiative in quantifiable measures.

Still, Bethel would like to be able to report its successes in deeper, more accurate and more comprehensive numbers, mainly so that they can influence public policy and help other groups get started. "In order to heighten the opportunity," says Nelson, "we need to have a research and evaluation arm that collects data and looks at the impact that we are having. We have always done 'Lessons Learned' on troubled programs, but we haven't always done it on the ones that worked." A recent grant will allow Bethel to hire consultants to study the problem of quantifying Bethel's effect on its community.

Because of the way it has grown, the Bethel New Life effort has taken a variety of organizational structures to fit different needs. The main structure is permanent and formal: a not-for-profit community development corporation, independent of its founding church, with a board of trustees and a board of advisors. That corporation, in turn, is part of several other consortia, including Westside Isaiah and the West Garfield Empowerment Zone Collaborative. A number of Bethel New Life's projects, such as the recycling business, are set up as subsidiaries. Others are joint ventures with other organizations, or straight contractual relationships. Some relationships, such as those with the organizations that provide healthcare to the people in Bethel's senior programs, have no formal shape at all.

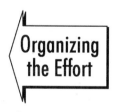

Organizing the Effort

I tell people to just start somewhere. The next steps will come.

Bethel has evolved away from "trying to do everything ourselves," as Nelson puts it, and toward partnerships. Experiences with attempting to be a healthcare provider in the late 1980s and early 1990s convinced Bethel that there are some things that are better left to others.

Bethel New Life allows us to see how the fight to rebuild community can take many different shapes—in fact, it must take a different shape for every community. And yet, though the shape on the surface may be different, there is much about the work that is deep and constant—a reaching back to roots for the true values of the community, gathering the strengths of the whole community, and creating a future together based on those strengths and values. "That's how Bethel evolved," says Nelson, "but it doesn't have to take that long. I tell people to just start somewhere. The next steps will come. The evolution will happen. If you try to be global and wait until you can do everything at once, you can end up waiting too long."

Mesa County, Healthy Community 2000

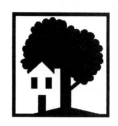

I f you've ever driven Interstate 70 from, say, Salt Lake City to Denver, you've been in Mesa County, and you have driven through Grand Junction, its county seat. Mesa counts 100,000 citizens peppered across the sprawling expanse of the western slope of the Rockies, tucked into small cities and towns, and spread across the great mesas, precipitous canyons, and broad, peaceful valleys.

It's a land of awe-inspiring vistas. Peer from a clifftop down Grand Valley, catch the glint of the sun off the Colorado winding through it. Despite the green of the bottom land and the forests on the mesas, it's not a lush landscape, and it has never been an easy place to live.

Ninety percent of the people live in this one valley. Very few of them are African-American, Asian, or Native American. Only 10 percent are Hispanic. As in most of the West, much of the land here is controlled by the federal government, and the economy is based on farming, mining, and tourism.

A paradise, an outsider might think. Far from the madding crowd. No smog. No gangs, no gunshots or sirens in the night. No traffic jams. No stress. No crack dealers on the corner. No slums, no decaying tenements with lead in the paint and in the pipes. What could be healthier?

But a closer look shows that Mesa County could, indeed, be healthier. Most people here live alone—those 100,000 people live in 80,000 households. Income levels are 17 percent below the state average, unemployment rates one-quarter higher, poverty levels one-third higher. There are homeless people. There are people dying of AIDS (78 so far), yet people think of AIDS as something that "can't happen here." Mesa's incidence of high blood pressure is 22 percent higher than the state average, and high cholesterol 17 percent higher. In a place that looks like Marlboro Country, 22 percent of adults smoke (34 percent of the young men) and most people do no regular exercise. Among 12th-grade girls, 38 percent will admit to having used marijuana in the past year, 15 percent to having used hallucinogens—and kids say there is "nothing to do around here."

Organizing the Effort

By early 1992, two groups had set out to improve the situation. A dental task force was trying to figure out how to help poor residents take better care of their teeth. And the county Health Department had begun a community health assessment. In May, the two got together and formed the nucleus of what would become the "Initiating Committee" of a Healthy Community 2000 effort. They applied to the Colorado Trust to be part of the Colorado Healthy Community Initiative. In November, they were chosen as one of the dozen "Cycle One" participants from around the state.

Convening the Community

By spring 1993 they were ready for a "Stakeholders Kickoff" meeting. National Civic League (NCL) facilitators helped the Initiating Committee work out who to invite. As in most such efforts, they sought demographic diversity. They also sought a balance between "ordinary people" and those who controlled most of the resources and political processes in the county. And they tried to leaven the process with people who had never taken part in anything like it.

Creating a Shared Vision

Larry Chynoweth of the Mesa County Health Department attributes the success of what followed to two factors: "First, an effort has been made throughout the process to include all the players. Second, vision is primarily a spiritual quality. To form a common vision, the souls of the people must be touched." Of the 140 souls invited to the kickoff meeting, 90 showed up to answer one essential question: "If I had a dream for my community, it would be . . ."

Assessing Current Realities and Trends

The stakeholders worked through the NCL Civic Index, grading the county in 18 areas spread across the economy, the environment, education, health, and social or civic capacities.

Some of their judgments stirred up controversy. Based on arrest statistics, they gave the county a "D" in public safety—which the sheriff took as a personal insult, a disparagement of his ability to do his job. A new reporting procedure, it turned out, added some minor crimes that had been overlooked before, causing a bump in the statistics. In the end, the sheriff did not quit the community-building effort, but instead became more involved. Chynoweth cites this problem as an example of "a shortcoming of these quick community evaluations—you have to be really careful with statistics."

Consensus does not always mean unanimity.

Perhaps surprisingly, the one large local community agency that has shunned the effort is the largest school district, which cares for more than 90 percent of the students in the county. According to

Chynoweth, "some of the recreation projects we have considered would involve building new combination schools–community centers, but we have had great difficulty getting any decision-makers from the school district at the table. The superintendent is a great proponent of community-based schooling, but he doesn't get involved. We have very little input from them—and we need it."

In such "rugged individualist" territory, it is perhaps not surprising that some of the invited stakeholders became disgruntled with the process and stayed disgruntled. Consensus does not always mean unanimity. "We don't want people coming in here and telling us what to do," states Chynoweth. "We all have the sanctity of our own projects and agencies, and it's hard for people to let go of their own ideas." Still, "I thought we were really successful in getting people to lay down their special issues . . . as long as we're just talking. But when it comes down to who gets the money, the old ugly stuff crops up again. . . . I don't think we solved [everything] but we have had some success in working through it."

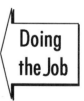

Action Planning

But by March 1994, when the community celebrated the end of the planning process, they did have a consensus. The stakeholders had developed a 10-year plan of action, focused on five specific new community assets:

- a Y.M.C.A or similar community recreation center

- a Community Master Development Plan

- a Transportation Awareness and Action Plan

- a community electronic network

- a Civic Forum

Doing the Job

Of these five, people are already working on the electronic network, the master plan, and the Civic Forum.

The electronic network is up and working in the form of a Web site (http://www.tapirback.com/mesa-co/) put up by Tapirback Enterprises, a small firm run by a pair of refugees from Los Angeles. The Web site features civic events, maps of the area, information about resources, and lots of pretty pictures of the area's breathtaking scenery.

The governments of the area (the county, cities, and special districts) are working out an area master plan with input from the Healthy Community 2000 assessments and the Civic Forum.

In many ways the Civic Forum turned out to be one of the most important concrete outcomes of the effort. A neutral nonpartisan organization that allows a civil debate, it is already meeting regularly, buoyed by a $100,000 two-year grant from the Colorado Trust. The Civic Forum has selected a board of directors, applied for nonprofit status, hired staff, and begun its own strategic planning. Its method is to pick a subject that the surveys have shown is important to the citizens—such as affordable housing, or growth, or teen violence—then hold hearings up and down the valley over a period of a month. The meetings are usually well attended. A VISTA volunteer is working with the group, researching the valley's transportation problem, which is deep—the valley has no public transportation at all.

They sought a balance between "ordinary people" and those who controlled most of the resources and political processes in the county.

Meanwhile, a second parallel effort had been unfolding. Sister Lynne Casey, head of St. Mary's Hospital, says, "I thought there were some natural synergies that could occur among the healthcare providers in the area. We had some conditions that were ideal for it: the size of the community, for one. The area was on a growth pattern, and a pattern of recovery from the downturns of the decade before. People were looking to the future, and we were outgrowing some of our traditional facilities and programs." When she arrived from Santa Monica, California, in 1990, she immediately set St. Mary's on a program of Total Quality Improvement, following the management precepts of the late W. Edward Deming. Part of that effort extended beyond the walls of St. Mary's, to their suppliers and partners, and to the institutions "upstream and downstream," for example, to Hilltop, a local rehabilitation hospital that got 80 percent of its business from St. Mary's. St. Mary's was the 600-pound gorilla of healthcare in the area, providing services for the whole region, and cooperation was not easy across such differences in scale. But the effort was exciting and different for the people of the area, bringing a demand for a kind of employee involvement and creativity that they had not experienced before.

There is a higher level of commitment and accountability now among those who took part.

In late 1992, Lynne Casey and Barbara Sowada, St. Mary's director of health education, went to a Peter Senge conference at Bretton Woods, looking for the next step. They encountered Bill Isaacs of the MIT Dialogue Project. He had a grant from the Robert Wood Johnson Foundation to use dialogue in an attempt to affect a social problem. They suggested that healthcare was a good place to start, and Grand Junction was an ideal community.

Their intent was to start a dialogue among their own staff, but when they returned, the associate director of Hilltop asked if Hilltop could be included in the effort. So they opened it up to all the healthcare providers in town. In all, the dialogue group held about 40 people, meeting two days per month, with the largest group from St. Mary's. After the first six months, which was covered by the grant, St. Mary's gathered a few partners to put on a second six months. St. Mary's paid a third of the costs, the Rocky Mountain HMO paid another third, and the rest was split among smaller participants.

The results were not unambiguous. There was some suspicion. "Some folks," says Sister Casey, "would say that St. Mary's must have something up its sleeve, since they are so committed to it. And I may have been naive. The process helped the synergy among the providers as I hoped it would, but it also surfaced deep fractures that were not healed by the process, such as people's belief systems about institutional agenda, about osteopathic versus allopathic medicine, about self-help, alternative, and traditional medicine. Still, I would do it again. There is a higher level of commitment and accountability now among those who took part."

And the effort did bear real fruit. During the dialogue project, one question came up repeatedly: What could we be doing differently to make a difference for people's health here in Mesa County? At St. Mary's invitation, a coalition of healthcare providers and community organizations came together, determined to give the county a thorough physical. The 21 members of the coalition included the City of Grand Junction, every healthcare provider in the region, a local HMO, the United Way, the county Health Department, the state college, a school district, and the Chamber of Commerce.

Assessing Current Realities and Trends

This Community Health Assessment Task Force passed the tin cup in their own ranks (with St. Mary's kicking in the bulk of the money) and hired a research company to do the scutwork. Eleven focus groups pulled in more than 100 citizens, interviewers detailed the views of 55 "key informants" (people in touch with "risk environments," such as midwives, church leaders, allied health professionals, cops and judges, students and school officials), and called up more than 1,000 people to take them through a 20-minute, 126-question survey. They combined this with "secondary research," existing data from previous county sources, and from outside the county.

A lot of people won't sit and read—but take a video to a service club, or a high school, and you have an audience.

It took 15 months, but using these methods, the task force identified 14 major problem areas, and boiled those down to the county's top five health priorities:

- Teen pregnancy

- Transportation

- Recreation (an answer to the "there's nothing to do here" problem)

- Substance abuse

- Mental health (depression, dysfunctional families, suicide)

Once the survey was done in mid-1995, the coalition set out to publicize the results. They published a poster with lots of facts and the big picture, and a 138-page book with all the details. The local paper printed a summary. The task force's "greatest hit" was a 22-minute video based on their interviews with "key informants." "We used it all over the community," says Deedee Mayer, executive director of United Way for Mesa County, "to educate everyone in the community who would listen. People really commented on it. A lot of people won't sit and read—but take a video to a service club, or a high school, and you have an audience. It has been very useful."

True to the roots of the effort in dialogue, the poster and other materials did not emphasize the identities of the organizations behind the effort—no names, no logos.

Doing the Job

Then they set to work, putting together a local task force to deal with each priority. "We call them 'the trend benders,'" says Carolyn Bruce, director of planning at St. Mary's. "If trends continue the way they are going, we'll be a lot worse off."

The task force spent nine months broadening its reach beyond its original 21 providers. In four major community meetings, it hashed out action plans for each of the five areas. They ended up with seven major community initiatives and some twenty minor ones.

The five teams work autonomously, under a mandate to develop and carry out any action that they feel might produce measurable results. The task force provides volunteer facilitators and trainers to make the process as productive as possible. A 20-person coordinating committee helps all the teams and works as a "bridge" for crossover projects that might fall between the cracks.

"In a community this size, that's manageable," says Mayer. "The networks are very strong. There is a great esprit de corps to improve the quality of life here." She adds with a laugh, "As long as it doesn't cost anything. But it's easy to pull people together for the first stage of planning. We had bankers, and people from the Department of Social Services. We had all the major power bases—ranchers, the energy industry, even Club 20, a conservative organization that represents ranchers and such on the Western Slope. The majority leader of the state legislature and the president pro tem of the state senate are local, and we involved them. The only opposition was lethargy—and that ebbs and flows."

The task force plans to reassess its progress during 1997 and to repeat the health assessment in 1998. "As people work with the information and try to move forward to specific actions," says Mayer, "they see that it's not as neat and tidy as they originally saw it. Some people have trouble letting go."

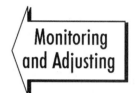

Monitoring and Adjusting

"The question," she continues, "is: how do we engage people outside the health or human service community over a long period of time. People say, 'I have a life. I can't go to meetings all the time. Yet we paid health and human services types lose touch, and that can be deadly."

"What we choose to do with this information will say a lot about where we go in the next decades. But I think we're going to see specific progress by the year 2000—we are already seeing some success in the teen pregnancy rate," says Mayer.

The difference between these two successive processes is striking—the one almost purely voluntary, inexpensive, and working by consensus, the other using paid researchers and consultants. The Healthy Communities 2000 planning effort cost approximately $15,000, according to Chynoweth, whereas the overall costs of the community health assessment was nearly $100,000. The health assessment effort went more smoothly than the planning effort—its goals were more confined, and the people involved shared a great deal of their professional background and assumptions. The planning effort was messier and more involved, "but I have more confidence in that process," says Chynoweth. "I am more comfortable with it." The health assessment actually involved more people than did the planning process, but only as respondents to surveys or members of focus groups.

Was one right and the other wrong? They served different needs. As a way to gather information, give the community a picture of itself, and urge people to think more deeply about their health, the health assessment worked wonderfully. As a way to mobilize citizens and get them involved in their own future, the planning effort and the resulting Civic Forums have been far superior.

Orlando, Healthy Communities Initiative

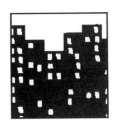

Marilyn King was frustrated, and she called her friend Linda about it. That's how it started. King was a longtime community volunteer, a former president of the Junior League, a trustee on the board of Orlando Regional Healthcare System, and chair of its community benefits committee. She had seen Orlando erupt from a sleepy live-oak-and-Spanish-moss Southern town into something entirely different. Because of the growth of the Kennedy Spaceport just to the east and Walt Disney World just to the southwest, Orlando had been one of the fastest-growing metropolitan areas in America in the seventies and eighties, exploding with retirees, high-tech, tourism, theme parks, and low-paying service industry jobs. Greater Orlando, now home to more than 800,000, was suffering all the maladies of nineties America, in its own special flavors.

Now it was 1993, and something was bugging King at a very deep level, something she could not quite name. She had just served on a pair of task forces dealing with children's issues and the juvenile justice system—"and it was clear that it wasn't working," she would say later. "We were not getting the results that we deeply needed to have, even though we had all these good professional people working on it, smart people, giving their best. But you know what they say: Insanity is doing the same thing over and over and expecting different results. We had to do something different. So I called Linda."

Linda Chapin listened carefully, busy as she was. She was chairman of Orange County, the county that contains Orlando, but, like King, she was also a former president of the Junior League. The next morning she called Marilyn from her cell phone in the car: "Listen, I just got a cancellation. Why don't you come in. We'll get some sandwiches and talk."

They talked. "I see people making these enormous efforts," she told Linda, "projects for every category of people and difficulties under the sun. But you know what? The problems don't stick to the categories. It doesn't work that way. We've got to try something new that cuts across the lines and brings these efforts together."

> We've got to try something new that cuts across the lines and brings these efforts together.

Chapin's advice? Spread the conversation. Marilyn should talk to John Haile, the editor of the *Orlando Sentinel.*

She did. "I made an appointment. I was afraid he would think I was batty." But he didn't. In fact, Haile had already been meeting with four or five friends, big players in town, about the same kinds of frustrations.

So they began to meet, just a few friends: Chapin, King, Haile, Diana Morgan from Disney, and Bill Mateer, who was a lawyer for Orlando Regional Healthcare and the *Sentinel* and a few others.

> ## Convening the Community

There was a clear sense of commitment to creating a greater community among the group, but there was not much agreement on what it would look like or how to get there.

These conversations, and a long series of lunches and coffees and tete-a-tetes that King had with every "power player" in town that she could get to, lasted for more than a year. "The groundwork that has to be laid, which seems a sort of soft issue, is absolutely critical," she now says of this time. "We could not have begun to make the systemic changes that we have without the buy-in of the people who ran those systems."

When they started, neither King nor any of those she spoke with were aware of any body of experience that could help them tackle these problems. But one day she picked up a healthcare journal that carried articles by Trevor Hancock and Len Duhl about the concept of a "Healthy City," which Duhl had been writing about since the 1970s, and which Hancock had pioneered in Toronto in the 1980s. To King, the ideas resonated perfectly with what she and her friends were attempting to do in Orlando. When she had lunch with Sharon McLearn, an executive at Orlando Regional Healthcare, she told her about the meetings, about the sense of frustration that they shared, about how stuck they felt—and about the articles she had read. McLearn said, "Let me tell you about something." Sharon had just finished a year of training in The Healthcare Forum's Healthy Communities Fellowship, along with Ted Hamilton, who was medical director of Florida Hospital. She had met, as faculty in the Fellowship, a range of experts from the Forum and the National Civic League. "I sent her boxes of materials," says McLearn now. King already knew The Healthcare Forum, and Orlando Regional was involved in their Daniel Yankelovich "What Creates Health?" study.

McLearn and Hamilton joined the meetings, by now grown to about 20 people. "The original group went around in a lot of circles," she says. "There was a clear sense of commitment to creating a greater community . . . but there was not much agreement on what it would look like or how to get there." King wanted to bring in a facilitator from The Healthcare Forum (THF) or the National Civic League (NCL). According to McLearn, the feeling of this high-powered group was, "We should be able to do this ourselves. We're smart people. We know what the problems are, we just need to do something about them." King's point of view? "We know what we think the problems are."

Eventually King prevailed. The group agreed to try a facilitator, just to see if it would work—and one person after another agreed to pay for a facilitator session.

The two organizations that they knew of offered somewhat different models for kick-starting a community process. The Healthcare Forum offered a town hall–style one-day event, whereas the National Civic League offered long-term facilitation. Given the choice, the group took both—a one-day event from The Healthcare Forum and long-term facilitation provided by the NCL.

Organizing the Effort

The facilitator was Gruffie Clough, who was both a senior associate at the Forum and a top facilitator with NCL—and the help paid off. "When we had some facilitation, we were able to home in on what we were trying to get out of this," says McLearn. Clough credits the group: "The key was that the Orlando people had really asked themselves excellent questions ahead of time." The group decided to call its effort the "Healthy Community Initiative of Greater Orlando" (HCI). They set out to create a formal Coordinating Committee by pulling in more people that they knew, the kind of active, community-oriented people that they felt could make a difference and bring some resources to bear.

When we had some facilitation, we were able to home in on what we were trying to get out of this.

They ended up with two dozen people at the first meeting in May 1994, including four additional former presidents of the Junior League, one of them the mayor of Orlando, Glenda Hood. The group included McLearn, plus the heads of several city departments, the Central Florida Healthcare Coalition (an employers' group), the school system, a local congregation, a bank, and a homeless coalition. Clough says, "They went from a handful of dreamers and visionaries to four handfuls of instigators whose job it was to plan the planning process."

Convening the Community

This group had four tasks:

1. To come up with a definition and a mission for the effort. After much debate, they created a working version of an overall goal—an Orlando that was a great place to raise kids would be a great place for everyone.

2. To select stakeholders to take part in the far larger planning process.

3. To form committees of support and infrastructure, such as outreach, research, logistics, and fundraising.

4. To plan the stakeholders' kickoff meeting. When they set the date for the first three-hour meeting of the stakeholders, they picked October, only five months in the future.

It was thought-provoking, educational and maybe a little threatening.

"It was very exciting work," says Clough now of those meetings every month from May to October, "and very productive, because of the very consistent work of the leadership, especially Sharon and Marilyn. It was thought-provoking, educational and maybe a little threatening. These two dozen people were undergoing some . . . changes in attitude, learning systems thinking, changes in perceptions. They couldn't make the decisions in the old adversarial ways—taking votes, declaring winners and losers—or have the same outcome, with the same old stakeholders. These were powerful people. If these people didn't experience a change, we had no hope of changing the city later on. That's what I have experienced in this kind of work: If the leaders don't change, the community doesn't. These leaders had to model the behaviors that they wanted for the citizens. If they showed up late, didn't listen well, and jumped to conclusions, that's what they would model. That was one reason this phase was so important, and one reason Orlando was so successful, along with Marilyn and Sharon and the backing of the hospitals. Marilyn did hours and hours of behind-the-scenes work, phone calls, listening to people. In other communities I have seen a lot people cut a lot of corners, a lot of "iffie" commitment. In Orlando, they committed to it and they didn't turn back. They just did this right from the very beginning."

The response stunned the committee. Almost everyone said yes.

After working with Clough to get a sense of where they wanted to go and what kind of people would need to be involved, they set out to gather them. Haile, of the *Sentinel,* kept pushing them to go beyond "the usual suspects." "It became an article of belief that we must not build a committee of people that we knew," says Sidney Green, a Coordinating Committee member and herself a "usual suspect," as a former president of the Junior League. "That became a real challenge."

The first attempt showed Haile's point. "Everybody made lists," said McLearn. "They were almost all upper-middle-class, professional, white, 35 to 65 years old, and educated. There was this 'Aha!' moment when we realized that we were traveling in pretty homogeneous circles."

For a second pass, the committee divvied up the economic sectors and demographic groups that would have to be represented, such as tourism, the service industry, Hispanics, African-Americans, and older people. Each member of the task force picked a group, did some research, asked around, thought about it, and came up with some names—more than 600 in all, stuck up on the walls on Post-Its. They put them in a database, categorizing them by race, marital status, age, location, and so forth. The one group they had trouble getting involved with (and still do) was Hispanics. In a series of meetings, they pared the list. They couldn't seem to get below about 164—but that would be fine, because, they assumed, at least half of the people would decline the invitation to so much work and trouble. Then they would do a second mailing to "fill in the holes." Eighty would be a nice number.

They were wrong. They sent out a mailing, a nicely designed, well-written, four-page brochure called "Destination: Imagination" that invited the reader to imagine a "safe, healthy, and rewarding" Orlando, and spelled out exactly what would be asked of the stakeholders, from the dates of the meetings to the fact that the process might become difficult and might require patience. The cover letter, which listed the names of the committee down one side, invited the receiver to attend. A response card had check-off boxes for accepting or declining the invitation and for requesting help with child care, transportation, getting time off work (the meetings would begin at 4 o'clock in the afternoon) or other problems.

The response stunned the committee. Almost everyone said yes. No second mailing was needed.

The stakeholders' agenda was ambitious—11 meetings over eight months to create a vision, build teams, assess the environment, identify leverage points and key performance areas, and map out

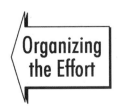

Organizing
the Effort

actions. They would need support. Orlando Regional Healthcare loaned the services of McLearn and her secretary, part-time, as staff for the effort. McLearn and the Coordinating Committee asked both organizations and individuals for help with everything from the consultants' fees to meeting space, copying, mailings, and even food for the meetings.

The committee approached the Orlando Foundation for help, but it didn't work out, for the very reasons that the Healthy Community Initiative was so powerfully different from the usual efforts: It cut across categories, it had no clearly defined outcome, it would not even know what it was planning to do until it had listened hard to everyone in town. "We could not fit into their boxes," says King.

The major players, such as the two hospital systems and several large employers, gave most of the support. Yet all this help was kept very much in the background. No one got their logo on anything. No one got touted as a sponsor. "It was important that we not look 'fat,'" says Green. Organizations and individuals would be publicly acknowledged for their help, but with an egalitarian touch. No one got more credit for giving more. In the initiative's vision publication, everyone from Orlando Regional Healthcare and Disney to the bakery that donated a tray of doughnuts would be listed—in alphabetical order. King had seen far too many "hospitals touting themselves as the leaders of Healthy Communities efforts. We went out of our way to de-emphasize the hospitals. This was about people, not about promoting institutions." This reflected King's deep values, her commitment to "doing the right thing." When Orlando Regional's CEO had asked her to take on the community benefits committee, she told him that she wasn't interested unless "community benefits" could mean more than marketing, and more than meeting the letter of the not-for-profit tax laws.

But it was more than the right thing. It was tactically smart. "There's no one's name on it," says McLearn. "In fact, a lot of the big players in town are involved, but if it belongs to anyone, it won't be as successful. Everyone has some baggage. People will think that you're doing it for the credit, that you're controlling it."

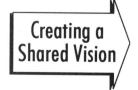

Creating a
Shared Vision

A few organizations have offered help, then withdrawn it when they discovered that they could not put their logo on it—but only a few.

When the stakeholders finally met, they set right to their tasks, with the help of The Healthcare Forum's one-day event, with such outsiders as Trevor Hancock of Toronto, the NCL's Tyler Norris, healthcare futurist Leland Kaiser, pollster Daniel Yankelovich, and Kathryn Johnson of The Healthcare Forum. The first task was to discover a common vision, a ground on which to build everything that would come after. Hancock reminded them that they all carried a vision of a healthy community in their heads, and invited them to search it out and share it, draw it, talk about it. When they had worked out a rough draft of the collective vision, a vision committee took over the work.

Over several months, starting in February 1995, the stakeholders conducted 30 focus groups of Orlando residents, hearing the concerns and interests of such groups as West Orange residents, Housing Authority residents, immigrants, young adults, gays and lesbians, Christian religious leaders, and owners of small businesses. That work shaped and refined the vision. One suggestion for change came from many different groups: When the vision document talked about what could be accomplished, many people heard nothing about personal responsibility. So the committee added an explicit statement on the importance of personal responsibility.

In the end, the vision contained 14 statements, on everything from the economy to children, from the arts, neighborhoods, and education, to interaction and security.

"It actually helps that we don't have the answers," says King. "We went to one small, very poor community. We held two focus groups for parents, 10 people in one, 11 in the other. Among other things, we asked them, 'What is the most important thing we could do to improve the lives of our children?' Now you and I could have made up a list a mile long, but 20 out of the 21 said something that would not have been on our list at all. They said, 'Teach us to read.'"

"When you listen to people, you build trust," says King. "If you have trust, you can disagree with people and still go forward. But you have to spend time building those relationships."

The stakeholders met about every three weeks in donated space in a local art museum, and talked over a donated dinner. Each time, they did specific activities to examine their own community, identify

> When you listen to people, you build trust, If you have trust, you can disagree with people and still go forward.

high-leverage areas, look for opportunities and threats, and explore their civic infrastructure.

"Eventually," says Clough, "we would ask, 'Now that you know it from a more diverse perspective, where are we going to make the biggest difference?' People gained new information and new insights. But one of the greatest outcomes of the process was the opportunity to build relationships.

"It was not easy at all. Many people, in fact most people, don't appreciate the value of process. They find it quite restrictive. Some people felt that they could identify the key areas at the very first meeting. Some people got frustrated. Some people spoke to me or Marilyn, some people quit coming. Some people were disruptive in the meeting. Some people said, 'Tell me again why we have to do this?' And I would say, 'Two reasons. One, if you look at all the research around human behavior, people do not change because of information. People change because of relationships. Two, if you don't understand it from all the perspectives, you won't be able to solve it.'"

Assessing Current Realities and Trends

The assessment phase went quickly, for a simple reason: They didn't reinvented the wheel. McLearn had recently done a similar study for Orlando Regional Healthcare. Combined with information brought to her by other members of the committee, it made for a comprehensive, numbers-filled, 100-page book of facts about Orange County's health and quality of life.

People do not change because of information. People change because of relationships.

To this they added the National Civic League Index, which measures a community's capacity for productive civic change. According to this index, Orlando was strong in leadership and philanthropy, but weaker in intergroup relationships and in civic education.

If the assessment were to mean anything, the numbers could not just sit in those 100 pages. They had to become real to the stakeholders. The presentations of these realities, in meetings through December 1994 and January 1995, were creative, different, and striking. One member of the research committee, assigned to transportation, took a video camera to an outlying district of the county, and recorded his efforts to take a bus to a specific address in Orlando. Another member of the research committee played the role of a single mother working for minimum wages, with so many dollars to go around, while other stakeholders played the part of the landlord, the grocery store, the daycare center, demanding payment. She managed to scrape by until suddenly her car broke down, and she was on the street. One stakeholder, a nurse with four kids, was homeless herself, and talked about how it happened and what it was like. A third research committee member had stakeholders pass around and collect playing cards to represent sexual contacts or shared needles. Some of the cards were marked as HIV carriers, and the infection spread through the group. Sidney Green says these presentations "had a powerful impact on all of us stakeholders."

Faced with these realities, the stakeholders set out to plan some actions. Several parameters arose from their discussion. They had not convened, they decided, to lobby Tallahassee or Washington. Instead, they would search for "key performance areas," points of maximum local leverage, areas where they could make a difference. That decision removed some problems from the table. Transportation, for instance, was indeed a problem, but most of the leverage and funds were controlled elsewhere.

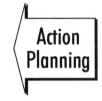

Action Planning

Another principle: They would build "initiatives," not "projects." The difference: They saw "projects" as the way well-meaning efforts usually turned out, focused on a single problem, with a particular method, particular sources of funds, and a distinct bureaucracy. HCI, in contrast, had to serve as the connective tissue bringing such narrow projects together in broad initiatives attempting to leverage change in whole segments of local society.

In the end, the stakeholders identified three "key performance areas":

- the need to strengthen families and support children

- the need to build community "connectedness" and promote collaborative efforts

- the need to accept, appreciate, and build upon diversity

The differences were like people looking at the same mountain through different lenses.

This last concern—a stand, essentially, against racism, sexism, and intolerance of all kinds—had a curious history. Almost every other concern showed up in substantial agreement across all different races, classes, and other groups, both in the focus groups and among the stakeholders. "The differences were like people looking at the same mountain through different lenses," as Sidney Green puts it. But on this one issue, there was stark division. Whites tended to dismiss racism as a major problem, whereas African-Americans put it at the forefront. In stakeholder discussions, some whites suggested that, in fact, the fight against racism was subsumed and honored in every conceivable initiative before them. But an African-American gave a different perspective: "That's why it's never dealt with, because it's never the main subject. It's always part of something else." In the end, the stakeholders came to consider diversity one of HCI's three main concerns.

For three more meetings, the stakeholders broke into small groups to hammer out action plans. The challenge was to get concrete, without breaking apart into a series of discrete "projects." "There are a million projects out there," says McLearn. "We want to attack the underlying issues. And we don't want to end up being the ones who are responsible for the community. Our goal is to get everyone in the community to see themselves as responsible for the community's future."

The group as a whole created five "Action Steps" (see box on next page).

That done, the stakeholders published a booklet with their findings in fall 1995, held a celebration, and participated in a three-hour video of the project prepared and aired by a local television station.

Then they cleared the decks for action. They had decided to turn the Healthy Community Initiative into a permanent organization, with a board, an endowment, and a building, to set the stage for fulfilling these plans.

> **Organizing the Effort**

"I didn't want to incorporate," says King. "I held off, kicking and screaming. We don't see ourselves as another agency, another provider, another entity in town. We are a connector. We bring people together—but we can't do that, in a substantive way, in a town this size, without full-time people. We have done the most comprehensive work for several years now on volunteer labor and part-time loaned people. You've got to have people who can give this their total focus." And you can't hire people, collect funds, and pay salaries unless you exist as a legal entity. So they incorporated as a 501c3 public benefit corporation, and began to gather a permanent board.

We have become very comfortable with ambiguity and uncertainty, very comfortable with not having answers.

Orlando Regional's "loan" of half of Sharon McLearn's time ended, and Sidney Green came on as full-time staff, a "director" with, at first, just a secretary. They were given a building, but it needed repairs and permits. All told, the reorganization took up the first half of 1996.

Action Steps

■ **Bring the various parties to the table to begin to create broad-based, community-wide, collaborative responses to significant community issues.**

- Focus early efforts on priorities identified by HCI stakeholders:
  - ▲ Community connectedness
  - ▲ Strengthening families and children
  - ▲ Diversity

■ **Develop a full spectrum of training opportunities for community trustees.**

- Include programs on facilitation, conflict resolution, mediation and leadership skills.

- Design leadership development program for grassroots leaders and untapped professionals.

- Work with schools to explore, develop and implement civic education curriculum.

■ **Increase the number of community stakeholders committed to the Healthy Community movement.**

- Launch a series of project-oriented community-building experiences.

- Develop communication vehicles to increase awareness of HCI goals, programs and concepts.

- Nurture media "civic journalism" role.

- Promote HCI programs and opportunities.

- Consider Neighborhood Watch approach.

■ **Facilitate the development of informational resources.**

- Ensure centralization and accessibility to the community.

- Integrate the latest technology.

■ **Provide celebration, recognition and revitalization programs for community trustees.**

Leland Kaiser, over lunch at the Orlando airport with Hamilton and Marilyn King, told them, "Of course, you've got to start by going to both of your institutions—Florida Hospital and Orlando Regional—and asking them to commit a million dollars." They did. And the institutions said yes. That kicked off a low-key, face-to-face campaign to get other institutions and employers in the area to kick into an endowment and a fund to pay the first year's operating expenses.

> **Doing the Job**

In the meantime, HCI's plans for action were on hold. Yet even during this breather, action did not stop. The spirit that HCI had stirred up in the community, and the awareness that it unleashed, began to turn up in projects that had no direct organizational connection to HCI, but were influenced by individual stakeholders. Two homeless programs stopped their turf competition and merged.

A "Collaborative Model Board"—an informal organization of public and private grant-giving agencies, chaired by King—began meeting to discuss how they could coordinate their grants to better serve the community. It brought major funders together with the mayor, the county chairman, representatives of state agencies (such as Health and Human Services), Disney, major foundations, and the head of the school system. "We're not telling anyone where to put their money," says King, "but we are beginning to evolve a shared vision of the community among those who fund things here."

County officials realized that it was futile to rebuild the physical infrastructure without dealing with the human element, the civic infrastructure.

The Citizens' Commission For Children dedicated $6 million to the "family support model." It declared that it would only fund organizations that were working collaboratively, because it is not effective to work with a child if you are not looking at the whole family—and it offered its grantees whatever help they needed to learn to work collaboratively with other providers. A number of local businesses began to take a hard look at their policies, searching for ways that they could be more "family friendly."

The county had already started a major "Targeted Communities" initiative dedicated to bringing a new direction to suffering communities by rebuilding the infrastructure. County officials realized that it was futile to rebuild the physical infrastructure without dealing with the human element, the civic infrastructure—and they invited the Healthy Community Initiative to work with them.

The next phase is to take those action plans to the next stage, to set goals, develop time lines, set benchmarks, and create mechanisms to monitor their progress in each area.

> **Monitoring and Adjusting**

McLearn feels that some of the action planning may have to be redone in more depth: "If you really want to attack these huge social problems, you can't create the action plan in three or four meetings with 20 people. You really have to reconvene a subset of the stake-holders, and bring some more people into the process, people with a stake in the situation, people with special experience, expertise, or information, and take them through a miniature version of the process to get to a consensus on the actions. The rush to get to actions and action plans—to 'do something'—causes people to end up at the same old things. We have enough momentum and cohesiveness now to take the time to do it fully."

For all of Orlando's rapid progress, it still takes a long view, sometimes, to see how quickly things are moving. One businessman told King that it was "the most exhilarating, and most frustrating" thing he had ever done. "People like me want to have an outline, we want to delegate the tasks and check them off." King admits that "it's not efficient in terms of time. It's about personal transformation. You have to change the whole way you get involved. Your value system has to permeate everything."

"There are still a lot of people who don't understand what we're trying to do," says McLearn. "People are a lot more comfortable with a project that has an endpoint, objectives, and a time line. To try to tell people that we're setting out on a journey with no guarantees is a lot harder. We have become very comfortable with ambiguity and uncertainty, very comfortable with not having answers. That's not how people typically do business.

"Marilyn and I sat in a meeting with a business leader one day who came right out and said, 'I really admire you folks, but I am quite concerned that you've taken on an impossible task. Look across society, morals are crumbling, things are falling apart. You're just going to get taught a very hard lesson.'"

"Everybody says it's an impossible job, it can't be done," says King. "We feel that we don't know how to do it, but it must be done."

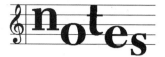

Conclusion

Conclusion

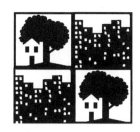

Having read the four case studies at the end of this workbook, you may get the feeling that community collaboration is not a simple process. You are right! There are no easy solutions to the plights of communities around the globe, but to that same end there are examples—hundreds of examples—of groups welcoming the challenge to do something to remedy the troubles of their own communities. The authors of this workbook are unable to prescribe for you the "music" your community should make upon joining forces and mounting a concerted effort to improve the mass transit system in your downtown area. Instead it is up to you to decide the most appropriate strategy considering the resources to which you have access and the degree of commitment you can garner from your neighbors and friends.

You have read about the stellar efforts by the citizens of Aiken, South Carolina, as they formed the Infant Mortality Task Force in their community to begin to combat some of the problems they had faced for years. You have learned about the tremendous labor undertaken by the community in West Garfield Park, Chicago, to turn their neighborhood around against amazing odds. You have seen numerous examples from communities just like yours, from all over the continent, with dozens of challenges and seemingly insurmountable obstacles, that have overcome these impediments and begun to make incremental changes, slowly but surely improving the health of their communities.

It is time to get the ball rolling in your own backyard! Gather people together and let some of the community's collaborative leadership emerge. Remember that shared leadership representing the diversity of the community in all its glory is the key to community empowerment. Working together you must establish your shared vision via consensus—close your collective eyes and imagine your group's utopia—you can achieve it if you can envision it clearly When determining which steps to take, be sure to consider the incredible wealth of resources right inside your own town gate. Once you discover what is out there for the taking, your group needs to be strategic in planning its actions. Be specific and ensure the actions you plan are leverage-based. Without further ado, launch yourselves into action to do the job that needs to be done. Timing is important here. To make the most of your effort, be sure to take advantage of the synergy you have already created with your actions to date. As you proceed, keep your eyes wide open for any obstacles that may delay you or cause detours. If you monitor your progress, you will save time in the long run and be agile enough to make mid-course corrections. At each step, remember to return to the structure your group will have developed along the way. Before you know it, you too will be well on your way to calling your very own community an ideal home.

Your schools, businesses, and community events are unique. The plan you put into action will undoubtedly be like no other. Despite this, we like to think that the collective consciousness of community members, urban or rural, from north, south, east and west, can and will assist you in your efforts. These leaders have offered their secrets of success so that other leaders, like you, may prosper in their attempts to improve the quality of life in their communities. Take some and leave others, but be sure to continue sharing the secrets! And remember, it doesn't matter how you get there, you just need to begin today: Start creating your community's jazz.

Appendixes

Appendix A

Best Practices Survey Questions

The following survey is the tool that was distributed to communities across North America for the purposes of gathering "Best Practices" in collaboration to improve health.

Organizing the Effort: Create processes for decision making, developing and sharing leadership and accountability, and communication.

> Please consider the following in your answer: How are you sharing leadership and accountability? Which processes have you put in place for joint decision making? Which communication vehicles do you use? How do you know you have been successful? Do you have any suggestions for other communities in adapting this series of actions or practices to their effort?

Convening the Community: Gain the commitment of stakeholders from multiple sectors and organizations to both the process of collaboration and to the desired population health outcome(s) of the effort.

> Please consider the following in your answer: How did you include diverse stakeholders? Which event, person or organization catalyzed the effort? How did you assess community readiness? What did you do to ensure credibility? How do you know you have been successful? Do you have any suggestions for other communities in adapting this series of actions or practices to their effort?

Creating a Shared Vision: Using a consensus-based process, develop a clear and compelling picture of the community's future health that serves as a guide for collaboration and collective action.

> Please consider: Which process did you use to develop your shared vision? How do you continually recreate and refine the shared vision? How do you know you have been successful? Do you have any suggestions for other communities in adapting this series of actions or practices to their effort?

Assessing Current Realities and Trends: Using a variety of methods, gain a clear understanding of the key dimensions and determinants of health.

> Please consider: How did you choose what to measure? Are you measuring assets as well as needs? How do you capture multiple points of view? How do you know you have been successful? Do you have any suggestions for other communities in adapting this series of actions or practices to their effort?

Action Planning: Design a detailed, high-leverage, strategic plan for collaborating to address the shared vision.

Please consider: Which process did you use to identify shared priorities? How did you address the need for short- and long-term actions? How do you know you have been successful? Do you have any suggestions for other communities in adapting this series of actions or practices to their effort?

Doing the Job: Using the action plan as a guideline, take actions that are timed and coordinated so they yield the greatest returns.

Please consider: How do you link doing with vision, assessment, action planning and outcomes? How do you select high-leverage actions? How do you prioritize resource allocation? How do you know you have been successful? Do you have any suggestions for other communities in adapting this series of actions or practices to their effort?

Monitoring and Adjusting: Measure the success of the effort in achieving its goals cost- and time-effectively (the ends), and measure the success of the process of collaboration itself (the means).

Please consider the following in your answer: How do you determine shared benchmarks and outcomes? What have you done to ensure you are monitoring progress from the outset? Which steps do you take to apply what you learned to immediately improve the effort? How do you know you have been successful? Do you have any suggestions for other communities in adapting this series of actions or practices to their effort?

Appendix B

Capacity Inventory

The following is the Capacity Inventory referred to in the chapter on assessing current realities and trends. Its purpose is to maximize your understanding of all of the assets within your community.

Hello. I'm with (your partnership's name). We're talking to local people about their skills. With this information, we hope to help people contribute to improving the well-being of our neighborhood. May I ask you some questions about your skills and abilities?

Part I—Skills Information

Now I'm going to read to you a list of skills. It's an extensive list, so I hope you'll bear with me. I'll read the skills and you just say "yes" whenever we get to one you have.

We are interested in all your skills and abilities. They may have been learned through experience in the home or with your family. They may be skills you've learned at church or in the community. They may also be skills you have learned on the job.

Health

❑ Caring for the Elderly

❑ Caring for the Mentally Ill

❑ Caring for the Sick

❑ Caring for the Physically Disabled or Developmentally Disabled

   (If "yes" was answered to items 1, 2, 3 or 4, ask the following)

Reprinted with permission from John McKnight and John Kretzmann, ABCD Institute, Institute for Policy Research, Northwestern University, Evanston, IL, 60208. Taken from *Building Communities from the Inside Out. A Path Toward Finding and Mobilizing a Community's Assets.* (Evanston, IL: 1993).

Now, I would like to know about the kind of care you provided.

❏ Bathing
❏ Feeding
❏ Preparing Special Diets
❏ Exercising and Escorting
❏ Grooming
❏ Dressing
❏ Making the Person Feel at Ease

Office

❏ Typing (words per minute _____)
❏ Operating Adding Machine/Calculator
❏ Filing Alphabetically/Numerically
❏ Taking Phone Messages
❏ Writing Business Letters (not typing)
❏ Receiving Phone Orders
❏ Operating Switchboard
❏ Keeping Track of Supplies
❏ Shorthand or Speedwriting
❏ Bookkeeping
❏ Entering Information into Computer
❏ Word Processing

Construction and Repair

❏ Painting
❏ Porch Construction or Repair
❏ Tearing Down Buildings
❏ Knocking Out Walls
❏ Wallpapering
❏ Furniture Repairs
❏ Repairing Locks
❏ Building Room Additions
❏ Tile Work
❏ Installing Drywall and Taping
❏ Plumbing Repairs
❏ Electrical Repairs
❏ Bricklaying & Masonry

(Stop here if no affirmative response by this point.)

❏ Cabinetmaking
❏ Kitchen Modernization
❏ Furniture Making
❏ Installing Insulation
❏ Plastering
❏ Soldering/Welding
❏ Concrete Work (sidewalks)
❏ Installing Floor Coverings
❏ Repairing Chimneys
❏ Heating/Cooling System Installation
❏ Putting on Siding
❏ Tuckpointing
❏ Cleaning Chimneys (chimney sweep)
❏ Installing Windows
❏ Building Swimming Pools
❏ Carpentry Skills
❏ Roofing Repair or Installation

Maintenance

❏ Window Washing
❏ Floor Waxing or Mopping
❏ Washing and Cleaning Carpets/Rugs
❏ Routing Clogged Drains
❏ Using a Handtruck in a Business
❏ Caulking
❏ General Household Cleaning
❏ Fixing Leaky Faucets
❏ Mowing Lawns
❏ Planting and Caring for Gardens
❏ Pruning Trees and Shrubbery
❏ Cleaning/Maintaining Swimming Pools
❏ Floor Sanding or Stripping
❏ Wood Stripping/Refinishing

Food

❐ Catering

❐ Serving Food to Large Numbers of People (more than 10)

❐ Preparing Meals for Large Numbers of People (more than 10)

❐ Clearing/Setting Tables for Large Numbers of People (more than 10)

❐ Washing Dishes for Large Numbers of People (more than 10)

❐ Operating Commercial Food Preparation Equipment

❐ Bartending

❐ Meatcutting

❐ Baking

Child Care

❐ Caring for Babies (under 1 year)

❐ Caring for Children (1 to 6)

❐ Caring for Children (7 to 13)

❐ Taking Children on Field Trips

Transportation

❐ Driving a Car

❐ Driving a Van

❐ Driving a Bus

❐ Driving a Taxi

❐ Driving a Tractor Trailer

❐ Driving a Commercial Truck

❐ Driving a Vehicle/Delivering Goods

❐ Hauling

❐ Operating Farm Equipment

❐ Driving an Ambulance

Operating Equipment and Repairing Machinery

❐ Repairing Radios, TVs, VCRs, Tape Recorders

❐ Repairing Other Small Appliances

❐ Repairing Automobiles

❐ Repairing Trucks/Buses

❐ Repairing Auto/Truck/Bus Bodies

❐ Using a Forklift

❐ Repairing Large Household Equipment (e.g., refrigerator)

❏ Repairing Heating and Air Conditioning System
❏ Operating a Dump Truck
❏ Fixing Washers/Dryers
❏ Repairing Elevators
❏ Operating a Crane
❏ Assembling Items

Supervision

❏ Writing Reports
❏ Filling Out Forms
❏ Planning Work for Other People
❏ Directing the Work of Other People
❏ Making a Budget
❏ Keeping Records of All Your Activities
❏ Interviewing People

Sales

❏ Operating a Cash Register
❏ Selling Products Wholesale or for Manufacturer (If yes, which products?)
❏ Selling Products Retail (If yes, which products?)
❏ Selling Services (If yes, which services?)
❏ How have you sold these products or services?

(If yes, check all that apply.)

    ❏ Door to Door

    ❏ Phone

    ❏ Mail

    ❏ Store

    ❏ Home

Music

❏ Singing
❏ Play an Instrument
   (Which instrument?) _____

Security

- ❐ Guarding Residential Property
- ❐ Guarding Commercial Property
- ❐ Guarding Industrial Property
- ❐ Armed Guard
- ❐ Crowd Control
- ❐ Ushering at Major Events
- ❐ Installing Alarms or Security Systems
- ❐ Repairing Alarms or Security Systems
- ❐ Firefighting

Other

- ❐ Upholstering
- ❐ Sewing
- ❐ Dressmaking
- ❐ Crocheting
- ❐ Knitting
- ❐ Tailoring
- ❐ Moving Furniture or Equipment to Different Locations
- ❐ Managing Property
- ❐ Assisting in the Classroom
- ❐ Hair Dressing
- ❐ Hair Cutting
- ❐ Phone Surveys
- ❐ Jewelry or Watch Repair

Are there any other skills you have that we haven't mentioned?

Priority Skills

1. When you think about your skills, which three things do you think you do best?

   a)

   b)

   c)

2. Which of all your skills are good enough that other people would hire you to do them?

   a)

   b)

   c)

3. Are there any skills you would like to teach?

   a)

   b)

   c)

4. Which skills would you most like to learn?

   a)

   b)

   c)

Part II—Community Skills

Have you ever organized or participated in any of the following community activities? (Please check all that apply.)

❏ Boy Scouts/Girl Scouts
❏ Church Fundraisers
❏ Bingo
❏ School-Parent Associations
❏ Sports Teams
❏ Camp Trips for Kids
❏ Field Trips
❏ Political Campaigns
❏ Block Clubs
❏ Community Groups
❏ Rummage Sales
❏ Yard Sales
❏ Church Suppers
❏ Community Gardens
❏ Neighborhood Organization
❏ Other Groups or Community Work?

Let me read the list again. Tell me in which of these you would be willing to participate in the future. (Please check all that apply)

(Repeat list above.)

Part III—Enterprising Interests and Experience

A. Business Interest

1. Have your ever considered starting a business?
   Yes _____   No _____

   If yes, what kind of business did you have in mind?

   _____

2. Did you plan to start it alone or with other people?
   Alone _____ With others _____

3. Did you plan to operate it out of your home?
   Yes _____   No _____

4. Which obstacle kept you from starting the business?

   _____

B. Business Activity

1. Are you currently earning money on your own
   through the sale of services or products?
   Yes _____   No _____

2. If yes, which are the services or products do you sell?

3. Whom do you sell to?

4. How do you get customers?

5. What would help you improve your business?

Part IV—Personal Information

Name _____

Address _____

Phone _____

Age _____
(If a precise age is not given, ask whether the person is in the teens, 20s, 30s, etc.)

Sex F_____ M_____

Thank you very much for your time.

Source _____

Place of Interview _____

Interviewer _____

Appendix C
Logic Model

Assumptions/Hypotheses
(Principles and Givens)

Why Engage Communities in Change

1. People should have access to healthcare, which encompasses more than medical care.
2. Health is a community issue, and communities will form partnerships to resolve healthcare problems.
3. Healthcare is predominantly purchased, delivered and consumed in local communities.
4. Communities can influence and shape both public and market policy at local, state and national levels.
5. External agents, working in partnership with communities, can serve as catalysts for change.

Assumptions of the CCHMS Model

1. Expanding access to insurance coverage and healthcare services will improve health status.
2. Information on health status and systems is required for informed decision making.
3. Shifting revenues and incentives to primary care and prevention will improve health status.
4. Creating effective links among medical care, public health, and human services will improve health status.
5. Active participation by consumers, payers, and providers can facilitate building collaborative community support for the reform process.
6. Community foundations can serve as neutral conveners and bring diverse stakeholders to the table.
7. A planned change model from visioning to action can facilitate and guide the reform process.
8. Inclusive community leadership within a partnership entity can facilitate and sustain the reform process.
9. External technical assistance can supplement local expertise and facilitate the reform process.

Reprinted with permission from Comprehensive Community Health Models of Michigan and Harry Perlstadt, Ph.D., creator of the Logic Model.

Logic Model

Comprehensive Community Health Models of Michigan

A Required Input (Resources needed to accomplish goals)	B Planning Phase Activities (Months 1 to 18)	C Planning Phase Outcomes (At month 18)	D Implementation Phase Activities (Months 19 to 30)	E Implementation Phase Outcomes (Resources needed to accomplish goals)	F Long-Range Outcomes (At year 5)	G Desired Social Change
COMMUNITY 1. Broad based citizen involvement. 2. Neutral convener with fiduciary responsibilities. 3. Community support including in-kind and matching funds. 4. An inclusive decision making process drawing on local leadership and expertise. 5. A communication/information network, including media links. 6. Outreach mechanisms and feedback. **FOUNDATION** 1. Willingness to create effective partnerships with communities to help them identify and find quality, cost effective solutions to reform their healthcare system. 2. Planning guides, policy and research updates, parameters and overall direction. 3. Declining financial assistance for the process. 4. Expert consultants and technical assistance as needed. 5. Evaluation services and assistance as needed. 6. State and national networking and resource identification. 7. Training and leadership development.	**COMMUNITY** 1. Conducting community meetings to gain feedback and sanction decisions for community vision and planning. 2. Establishing and maintaining an inclusive community decision making process. 3. Establishing and maintaining a project administrative structure. 4. Establishing and maintaining ongoing workgroups to obtain community input and develop recommendations for the community health improvement plan. 5. Designing and implementing communication and outreach activities. **FOUNDATION** 1. Organizing network and consultant meeting for training and policy. 2. Providing technical assistance and training. 3. Providing evaluation services. 4. Providing project/partnership administration services. 5. Host legislative-executive briefings.	1. New relationships among stakeholders will provide a foundation for implementation activities. 2. Project structure and staff for operation, monitoring and evaluation the implementation phase are identified. 3. Community match and multi-stakeholder support is pledged. 4. Public support for plan is evident. 5. State, federal and market policy changes required for planning and implementation are identified. 6. Community Health Investment plan is developed, which incorporates a community vision and a systemic approach addressing • community healthcare decision making • community wide coverage • integrated health delivery system • integrated administrative structure • community-based health information system • community health assessment	1. Cultivating community leadership to carry vision and implement plans. 2. Providing leadership to establish organizational approaches including staff support to implement short-term recommendations and develop long-term plans. 3. Identifying and addressing financial, inter-organizational, and public policy barriers to achieving the recommendations. 4. Continuing to refine and improve communication and develop stakeholder and public support. 5. Continuing to refine and improve inclusive community decision making process. 6. Developing community and organizational capacity to respond to changes in the healthcare environment.	1. Document completion of short-term recommendations and lessons learned. 2. Evidence of a viable inclusive community decision making process, leadership, and administrative structures. 3. Complete a strategic plan to sustain and maintain the initiative through: • community-based fiscal support • changes in state, federal and market policy 4. Completed a long-term plan featuring a community vision and systemic approach including community priorities, activities and outputs leading to achieving • community healthcare decision making • community wide coverage • integrated health delivery system • integrated administrative structure • community-based health information system • community health assessment	**CORE OBJECTIVES:** 1. Comprehensive integrated health delivery system that elevates the roles of health promotion, disease prevention and primary care, integrates medical, health and human service systems. 2. Community wide coverage with access to affordable and appropriate care within a community defined basic health service plan with a strategy to include the under and uninsured. 3. Inclusive, accountable community healthcare decision making process. **SUPPORTING STRATEGIES:** 1. Periodic community health assessment, which utilizes community health profiles and other indicators of access, health status, system resource performance and behavioral risk. 2. Community-based health information systems, which include performance monitoring, quality and cost effectiveness measurement, accessible records and consumer satisfaction. 3. Community administrative process which supports focal points for health data, policy, advocacy and dispute resolution, plus coordination among payers and providers including co-location, in-service training and common intake forms.	1. Improved health status 2. Inclusive decision making 3. Increased efficiency of healthcare system

Appendix D
Sample Action Plan in Progress

This action plan in progress is used with permission from Memorial Hospital of South Bend, Indiana. It details the planning behind a hospital-school collaboration to improve student health.

Organization Name <u>New Prairie School-Memorial Project</u> **Date Plan Completed** _____

Activity Description (what is to be done)	Person(s) Responsible	Status (completed by)	Comments
1. Determine project outcomes and monitoring issues.	Barbara/Jeanine	Completed	
2. Meet with School Principals.	Mike	August 9	
3. Do a one-page summary describing our plan.	Rich/Mike	Completed	
4. Research population in the region and stats on free lunch.	Mike	Completed	
5. Finalize project budget.	Mike	Completed	
6. Contact Health Departments to request immunization clinics in the fall.	To Be Announced (TBA)	TBA	Set up a meeting Oct. 3 to discuss.
7. Seek School Board approval.	Mike	Completed	
8. Recruit/hire second nurse.	Jeanine	Completed	
9. Recruit/hire 5 health aids.	Jeanine	Completed	
10. Design Health Aid Orientation Plan.	Barbara/Jeanine	Completed	
11. Plan staff training.	TBA	August 15	
12. Plan methods to develop baselines for project outcomes.	TBA	October 2	
13. Plan Health Fair(s).	TBA		Fairs should take place betw. Oct. 31 & Nov. 15, 1996.
14. Update educational components of the curriculum.	Mike/Jim	Ongoing	Wrap up by June 15, 1997
15. Create survey form.	Jeanine/Barb	Completed	
16. Create cover letter.	Each Principal	TBA	
17. Develop publicity plan.	Mike	TBA	

Reprinted with permission of Memorial Hospital of South Bend, Indiana.

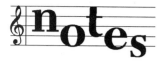

Glossary

Glossary

Action Team

Group of people focused on a particular part of the initiative who keep the activity and energy of the effort going.

Action Planning

Describes the partnership's goals for improving health, its objectives, and the high-leverage strategies and methods that it will use to address these goals and objectives.

Assessing Current Reality and Trends

Gathering of accurate, meaningful information about the key dimensions and determinants of health.

Assets

Useful or valuable tools that can lead to change.

Benchmark

A measured standard for comparison.

Collaborating

Exchanging information, modifying activities, sharing resources and enhancing the capacity of another for mutual benefit and to achieve a common purpose.

Communication

The exchange of thoughts, messages or information.

Cooperating

Exchanging information, modifying activities and sharing resources for mutual benefit and to achieve a common purpose.

Coordinating

Exchanging information and modifying activities for mutual benefit.

Coordinating Committee

Group of individuals who coordinate and oversee much of the collaborative process. They work closely with all stakeholders and staff members.

Core Process

A series of interrelated activities or events that convert inputs into results—in this case, successful collaboration outcomes.

Credibility

Trustworthy and reliable information.

Critical Mass

Crucial people or organizations.

Critical Success Factors

Actions and conditions that are essential for the development of each Core Process. Measures of effectiveness, efficiency and economy.

Doing the Job

The implementation phase of the effort.

Formal Leaders

Leaders within the community who are easily recognized by the public. They may be local elected officials, agency heads, service providers, prominent civic leaders, priests or rabbis.

Facilitator

Anyone who guides and accelerates the effort, initiative or program.

Grassroots

Individuals or society at a local level.

Healthier Communities

A term used internationally to describe a new way of thinking about complex health, social and environmental issues facing communities. The model focuses attention on whole systems rather than just the parts. The movement toward Healthier Communities began in 1986 when the World Health Organization (WHO) convened in Canada and created goals and programs (including the Ottawa Charter for Health Promotion and Healthy Cities) focusing on health promotion and disease prevention. In 1989, the U.S. Public Health Services worked with the National Civic League to develop the U.S. Healthy Cities Program. In 1990, the Healthier Communities philosophy was adopted by the American Hospital Association, Centers for Disease Control and many others.

Informal Leaders

Leaders who may not have a title, a conventional office or even a telephone. Informal leaders may run or work at a local store, may be the adopted "grandmother" of a neighborhood who sits out on her porch, or may be a drug dealer out on a street corner.

Metaprocess

The central Core Process, which serves as a foundation or structure to fortify the remaining Core Processes.

Monitoring and Adjusting

Continuous evaluation of the effort and implementation of improvement measures.

Networking
Exchanging information for mutual benefit.

Organizing the Effort
The Core Process that lies at the heart of the others. It acts as a Metaprocess, bridging gaps, and serves as the "sheet music" to fortify the remaining Core Processes.

Partnership
Forming a bond between two separate organizations in order to create change.

Primary Data
Information that does not exist within the community and needs to be gathered.

Secondary Data
Information that already exists in a community.

Shared Vision
A compelling statement of what one wants to create; the engine that drives strategies and gives them their force.

Stakeholder
Anyone who has a stake in an effort, initiative or program.

Steering Committee
A small subgroup of the collaborative effort that takes primary responsibility for the partnership's overall direction.

Synergy
The interaction of two or more agents so that their combined effect is greater than the sum of their individual effects.

Table Facilitator
Anyone who guides and accelerates the effort, initiative or program—often in a smaller group (e.g., around a table).

Resources

Bibliography by Workbook Section

Introduction

Flower, Joe. "Building Healthier Cities." *Healthcare Forum Journal.* (May-June 1993): pp. 48–54, 75.

Fuller, Jim. "Jazz as a Process of Organization Innovation." *Star Tribune.* (Minneapolis, MN: October 23, 1988).

—. The Healthcare Forum. *Developing Community Capacity. Module 1: Sustaining Community-Based Initiatives.* (San Francisco: January 1996).

—. The Healthcare Forum. *Healthier Communities Action Kit. Module 1: Getting Started.* (San Francisco: April 1994).

—. The Healthcare Forum. *Healthier Communities Action Kit. Module 4: Sustaining the Effort.* Chapter One—Sustainability: Concepts and Principles. (San Francisco, 1994). (Written by: Tyler Norris, 1919 - 14th Street, Suite 804, Boulder CO, (303) 444-3366).

Schwartz, Peter and Kelly, Kevin. "The Relentless Contrarian." *Wired.* (August 1996): pp. 116–120.

Senge, Peter M. *The Fifth Discipline: The Art and Practice of the Learning Organization.* (New York: Doubleday, 1990).

Organizing the Effort

Chavis, D. and Florin, P. *The Role of Block Associations in Crime Control and Community Development: The Block Buster Project.* Report to the Ford Foundation. (1987).

—. Center for Substance Abuse Prevention (CSAP). *Community Wheel.* (Georgia: 1994).

—. The Heathcare Forum. *Developing Community Capacity. Module 1: Sustaining Community-Based Initiatives.* (San Francisco: January 1996).

Wolff, Tom and Kaye, Gillian. *From the Ground Up! A Workbook on Coalition Building and Community Development.* AHEC/Community Partners. (Amherst, MA: 1991).

Convening the Community

Flower, Joe. "Building Healthier Cities." *Healthcare Forum Journal.* (May-June 1993): pp. 48–54, 75.

—. The Healthcare Forum. *The Community Forum Planning Manual.* (San Francisco: 1995).

—. The Healthcare Forum. *Developing Community Capacity. Module 1: Sustaining Community-Based Initiatives.* (San Francisco: January, 1996).

—. The Healthcare Forum. *Healthier Communities Action Kit. Module 1: Getting Started.* (San Francisco: April 1994).

Roberts, Micky. *Community Matrix.* (Clarkston Health Collaborative: Decatur, GA).

Wolff, Tom and Kaye, Gillian. *From the Ground Up! A Workbook on Coalition Building and Community Development.* AHEC/Community Partners. (Amherst, MA: 1991).

Creating a Shared Vision

—. The City Wide Planning and Improvement Agency. *Vision.* (North Philadelphia, PA).

—. The Healthcare Forum. *Communicating with Policy Makers. Module 2: Sustaining Community-Based Initiatives.* (San Francisco: 1996).

—. Healthy Roseville 2000 Forum, Roseville Healthy City Coalition. *Vision.* (Roseville, CA: October 1995).

Himmelman, Arthur T. "Collaboration for a Change: Definitions, Models, Roles and a Guide to Collaborative Processes." (September 1995).

Norris, Tyler. *Healthier Communities Action Kit. Module 4: Sustaining the Effort.* The Healthcare Forum. (San Francisco: 1994).

—. Partnerships for Tomorrow. *Vision.* (Burnsville, MN).

Senge, Peter M. *The Fifth Discipline: The Art and Practice of the Learning Organization.* (New York: Doubleday, 1990).

Stern, G. J. *Marketing Workbook for Nonprofit Organizations.* (St. Paul, MN: Amherst H. Wilder Foundation: 1990).

—. Truckee Meadow Regional Plan. *Vision.* (Reno, NV).

Wolff, Tom and Kaye, Gillian. *From the Ground Up! A Workbook on Coalition Building and Community Development.* AHEC/Community Partners. (Amherst, MA: 1991).

Assessing Current Realities and Trends

—. The Contra Costa County Health Services Department Prevention Program. *Developing Effective Coalitions—An Eight-Step Guide.* (Pleasant Hill, CA: 1994).

—. The Healthcare Forum. *Developing Community Capacity. Module 1: Sustaining Community-Based Initiatives.* (San Francisco: January 1996).

Lillie-Blanton, Marsha and Hoffman, Sandra C. "Conducting an Assessment of Health Needs and Resources in a Racial/Ethnic Minority Community." *Health Services Research.* (April 1995).Vol. 30, n.1, part II.

McKnight, John and Kretzmann, John. *Building Communities from the Inside Out. A Path Toward Finding and Mobilizing a Community's Assets.* (Evanston, IL: 1993).

Action Planning

—. The Healthcare Forum. *Developing Community Capacity. Module 1: Sustaining Community-Based Initiatives.* (San Francisco: January 1996).

—. The Healthcare Forum. *Strategic Simulation Series—The Community Builder: Strategies for Improving Quality of Life.* (San Francisco: 1996).

Senge, Peter M. *The Fifth Discipline: The Art and Practice of the Learning Organization.* (New York: Doubleday, 1990).

Wolff, Tom and Kaye, Gillian. *From the Ground Up! A Workbook on Coalition Building and Community Development.* AHEC/Community Partners. (Amherst, MA: 1991).

Doing the Job

Himmelman, Arthur T. *Collaboration for a Change: Definitions, Models, Roles and a Guide to Collaborative Processes.* (September 1995).

McKnight, John and Kretzmann, John. *Building Communities from the Inside Out. A Path Toward Finding and Mobilizing a Community's Assets.* (Evanston, IL: 1993).

Wolff, Tom and Kaye, Gillian. *From the Ground Up! A Workbook on Coalition Building and Community Development.* AHEC/Community Partners. (Amherst, MA: 1991).

Monitoring and Adjusting

Butterfoss, F.D., Goodman, R., and Wandersman, A."Community Coalitions for Prevention and Health Promotion." *Health Education Research: Theory and Practice.* (1993).

Himmelman, Arthur T. *Collaboration for a Change: Definitions, Models, Roles and a Guide to Collaborative Processes.* (September 1995).

Linney, J. A. and Wandersman, A. *Prevention Plus III.* U.S. Department of Health and Human Services. (Rockville, MD: 1991).

Wolff, Tom and Kaye, Gillian. *From the Ground Up! A Workbook on Coalition Building and Community Development.* AHEC/Community Partners. (Amherst, MA: 1991).

Illustrations

Many of the illustrations in the workbook were reproduced with permission from Ted Goff, Cartoonist, P.O. Box 22679, Kansas City, MO, 64113-0679.

Additional Resources

Following are resources of interest on Community Assessment, Collaboration and Coalition Building, and Healthy Communities. This list is by no means exhaustive but may be of use to the reader in pursuing additional information on community collaboration.

Community Assessment

Aday, L.A., et al. "Potentials of Local Health Surveys: A State of the Art Summary." *American Journal of Public Health.* (August 1981): pp. 835–840.

Bell, Roger, et al. Assessing Health and Human Service Needs. *Proceedings of the Louisville National Conference*, Louisville, 1976. (New York: Human Services Press, 1983).

Bloom, Bernard, Sr. "Assessing Health and Human Service Needs Concepts, Methods and Applications." *Community Psychology Series*: Vol. 8, chapters 11, 15, 16.

Dever, G. E. *Community Health Analysis.* (Rockville, MD: Aspen Publishers, 1991).

Goeppinger, J. and Baglian, A. J. "Community Competence: A Positive Approach to Needs Assessment." *American Journal of Community Psychology.* (1985):Vol. 13,pp. 507–523.

Hillery, George A. "Definitions of Community: Areas of Agreement." *Rural Sociology.* (June 1955):Vol. 20, pp. 111–123.

—. InterHealth Organizations. *A Guide to Community Health Needs Assessment Tools.* (InterHealth Organizations, September 1992).

Johnson, Donald E. *Needs Assessment Theory and Methods.* (Ames: Iowa State University Press, 1987).

Kimmel, Wayne A. *Needs Assessment: A Critical Perspective.* (U.S. Department of Health, Education and Welfare. December 1977).

McKnight, John and Kretzmann, John. *Getting Connected: How to Find Out About Groups and Organizations in Your Neighborhood.* (Evanston, IL: Center for Urban Affairs and Policy Research, Northwestern University, 1988).

—. National Civic League. *Civic Index Workbook.* (Denver: National Civic League, 1987).

Neuber, Keith A. *Needs Assessment: A Model for Community Planning.* (Beverly Hills: Sage, 1980).

Nix, N. "Community Reconnaissance Method of a Synthesis of Functions." *Journal of Community Development Society.* (1971):Vol. 11, pp. 62–69.

Rappaport, Julian. "In Praise of Paradox: A Social Policy of Empowerment Over Prevention." *American Journal of Community Psychology.* (1981):Vol. 9, pp. 1–25.

Rice, James A. "Community Health Assessment: The First Step in Community Health Planning." *American Hospital Association Hospital Technology Feature Report.* (1993):Vol. 12, (13).

Sanders, I. T. "The Social Reconnaissance Method of Community Study." *Research in Rural Society and Development.* (1985):Vol. 2, pp. 235–255.

Tonin, M. D. "Concepts in Community Participation." *International Journal of Health Education.* (1980):pp. 1–13.

—. U.S. Centers for Disease Control. *Community Resource Inventory.* (Atlanta, GA: 1988).

—. U.S. Centers for Disease Control. "Health Objectives for the Nation." *Morbidity and Mortality Weekly Report.* (July 12, 1991):PP. 49–51.

—. U.S. Centers for Disease Control. *A Guide to the Selection and Utilization of Selected Health Assessment and Planning Models to Improve Community Health and to Contribute to the Achievement of the Year 2000 Objectives* (Washington, DC: CDC, 1991).

—. United Way of America. *Needs Assessment: The State of the Art Guide for Planners, Managers, and Funders of Health and Human Care Services.* (Alexandria, VA: United Way of America, November 1982).

Voth, D. E. "Social Action Research in Community Development." (Community Development Research, 1979).

Collaboration and Coalition Building

—. American Medical Association. *Community Action: How to Work in Coalitions.* (Chicago: 1987).

Arkin, E. B. "Opportunities for Improving the Nation's Health Through Collaboration With the Mass Media." *Public Health Reports.* (1990):Vol. 105, pp. 219–223.

Benard, B. "Working together: Principles of Effective Collaboration." *Prevention Forum.* (October 1989):pp. 4–9.

Black, T. "Coalition Building: Some Suggestions." *Child Welfare.* (1983):Vol. 62, pp. 263–268.

Brown, C. *The Art of Coalition Building: A Guide for Community Leaders.* (New York: American Jewish Committee, 1984).

Butterfoss, F.D., Goodman, R., and Wandersman, A."Community Coalitions for Prevention and Health Promotion." *Health Education Research: Theory and Practice.* (1993).

Capozzalo, Gayle. "Collaboration as a Source of Strength." *Health Progress.* (November 1991):pp. 32–36.

Cassetta, Robin A. "Coalitions Bring Quality to Health Care Reform." *The American Nurse* (January 1993):p. 7.

Chapman, L. and Jurs, Jan. "Conducting Community Health Planning Through a Hospital Sponsored Coalition." *Journal of Health Education.* (March-April 1993): Vol. 24.

Chavis, D. and Florin, P. *Community Development, Community Participation.* (San Jose, CA: Prevention Office, Bureau of Drug Abuse Services, 1990).

Chrislip, David D. and Larson, Carl E. *Collaborative Leadership: How Citizens and Civic Leaders Can Make a Difference.* (San Francisco: Jossey Bass, 1994).

Coe, Barbara. "Open Focus: Implementing Projects in Multi-Organizational Settings." *International Journal of Public Administration.* (1988):Vol 11, pp. 503–526.

Cohen, D. "Collaboration: What Works?" *Education Week*. (March 1989):p. 13.

—. Contra Costa Health Services Department Prevention Program. *Developing Effective Coalitions—An Eight-Step Guide*. (Pleasant Hill: 1994).

Cook, Harold L. et al. "A Reexamination of Community Participation in Health: Lessons From Three Community Health Projects." *Family and Community Health*. (August 1988):pp. 1–13.

Couto, Richard A. "Promoting Health at the Grassroots." *Health Affairs*. (Summer 1990):pp. 144–151.

Croan, G. and Lees, J. *Building Effective Coalitions: Some Planning Considerations*. Westinghouse National Issues Center, Arlington, VA.

Dolan, T. C. "Board-CEO Relations: Collaboration and Community Service." *Trustee*. (1992):Vol. 43, p. 11.

Elelstein, M. "Building Coalitions for Sustainability: An Examination of Emergent Partnerships Addressing Environmental and Community Issues." Paper presented at the annual meeting of the Environmental Design Research Association, Boulder, CO.

Eng, E., Salmon, M., and Mullan, F. "Community Empowerment: The Critical Base for Primary Health Care." *Family and Community Health*. (1992):Vol. 15, pp. 1–12.

Feigherty, E. and Rogers, T. "Building and Maintaining Effective Coalitions." (Palo Alto, CA: Health Promotion Resource Center, Stanford University School of Medicine, 1990).

Feighery, E. and Rogers, T. "Building and Maintaining Effective Coalitions." Published as Guide No. 12 in the series, "How-to Guides on Community" (1989).

Gardener, John W. *Building Community*. (Washington, DC: Independent Sector, 1991).

Gittell, M. *Limits of Citizen Participation: The Decline of Community Organizations*. (Beverly Hills, CA: Sage, 1980).

Gray, B. "Conditions Facilitating Interorganizational Collaboration." *Human Relations*. (1985): Vol. 38, pp. 911–936.

—.The Healthcare Forum. *Community Forum Planning Manual* (San Francisco, 1995).

—.The Healthcare Forum. *Healthier Communities Action Kit. Module 4: Sustaining the Effort*. (San Francisco, 1994).

—.The Healthcare Forum. *Healthier Communities Action Kit. Module 4: Sustaining the Effort. Chapter One—Sustainability: Concepts and Principles*. (San Francisco, 1994). (Written by: Tyler Norris, 1919 - 14th Street, Suite 804, Boulder CO, (303) 444-3366).

—.The Healthcare Forum. *What Creates Health? Individuals and Communities Respond*. (San Francisco, 1994).

—.The Healthcare Forum/W.K. Kellogg Foundation. *Sustaining Community-Based Initiatives. Module One: Developing Community Capacity*. (1996).

Himmelman, Arthur T. "Community-Based Collaborations: Working Together for a Change." *Northwest Report*. (November 1990): p. 26.

Hord, S. "A Synthesis of Research on Organizational Collaboration." *Educational Leadership.* (February 1986):pp. 22–26.

Kaplan, M. "Cooperation and Coalition Development Among Neighborhood Organizations: A Case Study." *Journal of Voluntary Action Research.* (1986):Vol. 15(4).

LaBonte, R. *Health Promotion and Empowerment: Practice Frameworks #3.* (Toronto, Ontario, Canada: University of Toronto, Centre for Health Promotion, 1993).

Lappe, Frances Moore and DuBois, Paul Martin. *The Quickening of America.* (San Francisco: Jossey-Bass, 1994).

Mattessich, Paul W. and Monsey, Barbara R. *Collaboration: What Makes It Work?* (St. Paul, MN: Wilder Research Center, Amherst H. Wilder Foundation, 1992).

Miller, S. M. "Coalition Etiquette: Ground Rules for Building Unity." *Social Policy.* (Fall 1983):Vol. 14, pp. 47–49.

Minicucci, Stephen. *Healthy Boston: Mobilizing Community Resources Through Coalition Building: An Essay on the Idea and Implementation of Healthy Boston.* Cambridge, Massachusetts: Department of Political Science Massachusetts Institute of Technology. (November 1993).

Minkler, Meredith. "Health Education, Health Promotion and the Open Society: A Historical Perspective." *Health Education Quarterly.* (1989):Vol. 16, pp. 17–30.

Minkler, Meredith. Improving Health Through Community Organization. Edited by B. Rimer, F. M. Lewis and K. Glanz. *Health Behavior and Health Education.* (San Francisco: Jossey-Bass, 1990)

Minkler, Meredith. Improving Health Through Community Organization. Edited by B. Rimer, F. M. Lewis and K. Glanz. *Health Behavior and Health Education.* (San Francisco: Jossey-Bass, 1990)

Mizrahi, T. and Rosenthal, B. "Managing Dynamic Tension in Social Change Coalitions." *Community Organization and Social Administration: Advances, Trends, and Emerging Principles.* (New York: Haworth Press, 1992).

Oie, Melody and Recker, Diane. "Empowerment Through Collaboration: Implementing a Team Quality Assurance Model." *Journal of Nursing Care Quality.* (1992):Vol. 6, pp. 32–40.

Perlman, J. "Grassroots Empowerment and Government Response." *Social Policy.* (1979):Vol. 10, pp. 16–21.

Rich, R. "The Dynamics of Leadership in Neighborhood Organizations." *Social Science Quarterly.* (1980): Vol. 60(4), pp. 570–587.

Severson, David. "Collaboration, Cooperation, and Celebration." *Quality Progress.* (September 1992):pp. 63–65.

—. Voluntary Hospitals of America. *Sustaining Community Health Improvement Initiatives.* (Irving, Texas: VHA, 1995).

Wallerstein, Nina. "Powerless, Empowerment and Health: Implications for Health Promotion Programs." *American Journal of Health Promotion.* (1992):Vol. 6, pp. 197–201.

Wandersman, A. and Goodman, R. *Increasing the Effectiveness and Efficiency of Community Coalitions Through Basic and Action Research: A Concept Paper and Proposal.* Unpublished manuscript. (1990).

Winer, Michael and Ray, Karen. *Collaboration Handbook: Creating, Sustaining, and Enjoying the Journey.* (St. Paul, MN: Wilder Foundation, 1994).

Wolff, Thomas. *Coalition Building: One Path to Empowered Communities.* AHEC/Community Partners. (Amherst, MA: 1991).

Wolff, Tom and Kaye, Gillian. *From the Ground Up! A Workbook on Coalition Building and Community Development.* AHEC/Community Partners. (Amherst, MA: 1991).

Healthy Communities

—. American Public Health Association. *Healthy Communities 2000: Model Standards: Guidelines for Community Attainment of the Year 2000 National Health Objectives.* 3rd ed. (Washington, DC: 1991).

Arkus, Connie. "Enhancing Community Relations in a Health Reform Environment." *Trustee.* (July 1993):Vol. 46 (7).

Ashton, John. *Healthy Cities.* (Philadelphia: Open University Press, 1992).

Berkowitz, B. *Community Dreams: Ideas for Enriching Neighborhood and Community Life.* (San Luis Obispo, CA.: Impact Publishers, 1984).

Caudron, Shari. "Community Coalitions Influence Their Local Health Care." *Personnel Journal.* (September 1993):Vol. 72 (9), p. 114.

Conklin, Michele. "Improving Community Health Depends on Widespread Involvement." *Health Care Strategic Management.* (December 1994):Vol. 12 (12), p. 6.

Flower, Joe. "Building Healthier Cities." *Healthcare Forum Journal.* (May-June 1993): pp. 48–54, 75.

Flynn, Beverly C. *Healthy Cities in the United States.* Edited by J. Ashton. (Philadelphia: Open University Press, 1992).

Flynn, Beverly C. "Healthy Cities: A Model of Community Change." *Family and Community Health.* (1992):Vol. 15, pp. 13–23.

Gunderson, Gary. "Foundations Must Answer Community Health Needs." *Modern Healthcare.* (August 21, 1995):Vol. 25 (34), p. 110.

—. Healthy City Toronto. *State of the City Report Card.* Healthy Cities Toronto, (1993 with updates released in 1996). ADDRESS: 20 Dundas St. W., 10th Fl., Toronto, Ontario, Canada, M5G 2C2 (phone: 416-392-1086; fax: 416-392-0089) Contact: Lisa Salsberg.

Kovner, Anthony and Paul Hattis. "Benefitting Communities." *Health Management Quarterly.* (Fourth Quarter 1990):pp. 6–10.

Kroll, Steve. "Health Care Reform: Opportunities for Political and Community Advocacy." *Trustee.* (March 1992): Vol. 45 (3), pp. 8-9, 20.

Lillie-Blanton, Marsha and Hoffman, Sandra C. "Conducting an Assessment of Health Needs and Resources in a Racial/ethnic Minority Community." *Health Services Research.* (April 1995):Vol. 30 (1), part II, pp. 225–236.

Myers, Michael J. "The Community-Based Health Care Model: A Potential Silver Lining for South Dakota." *South Dakota Business Review.* (December 1993):Vol. 52 (21), p. 6.

—. National Civic League. *The Healthy Communities Handbook.* (Denver: National Civic League, 1993).

Oakley, Peter. *Community Involvement in Health Development: An Examination of the Critical Issues.* (Geneva: World Health Organization; Albany, NY: WHO Publications Center USA [distributor], 1989).

Orlikoff, James E and Totten, Mary. "Trustee Workbook: Assessing and Improving Your Community's Health." *Trustee.* (May 1995):Vol. 48 (5), SS1–SS4.

Patton, Robert D. and Cissell, William B. (Eds.). *Community Organization: Traditional Principles and Modern Applications.* (Johnson City, TN: Latchpins Press, 1990).

Pelletire, K. R., Klehr, N. C. and McPhee, S. J. "Town and Gown: A Lesson in Collaboration." *Business and Health.* (1988):Vol. 56, pp. 382–388.

Pitts, Terry. "The Illusion of Control and the Importance of Community in Health Care Organizations." *Hospital & Health Services Administration.* (Spring 1993):Vol. 38(1), pp. 101–109.

Reynolds, D. L. and Chambers, L. W. " Healthy Communications: Producing a Health Report (Infowatch) for Monitoring and Promoting Health in Local Communities." *Canadian Journal of Public Health.* (July-August 1992):Vol. 83 (4), pp. 271–273.

Sigmond, Robert M. "Back to the Future: Partnerships and Coordination for Community Health." *Frontiers of Health Services Management.* (Summer 1995) Vol. 11 (4), pp. 5–36.

Stundard, A., et al. "Mobilizing a Community to Promote Health: The Pennsylvania County Health Improvement Program." Edited by J. C. Rosen and L. J. Soloman. *Prevention in Health Psychology.* (1985).

Annotated Resources

Community Assessment

The primary goal of many community health initiatives is to improve the health and quality of life of the citizens of the community. Improvement implies movement from one point to another in a positive direction. Recognizing this movement requires the development of ongoing monitoring of a community health profile. This profile contains a set of key community health indicators that assist in setting priorities and documenting the success or relative success of a given project. Trends, both positive and negative, can be detected and tracked, helping to fine-tune community priorities and allowing appropriate action to be taken. Given time and resource constraints, your community will need to select the most relevant, useful and accurate measures relating to priority indicators. While there are few absolute standards for indicator selection, following certain guidelines will assist in developing the most effective community profile. There are a number of models that communities have used to create community health profiles. The following are examples of assessment models used by communities across the nation:

■ **Assessment Protocol for Excellence in Public Health (APEXPH)**

APEXPH is a self-assessment process for use by local health departments to assist them in better meeting the public health needs of their communities. The process is presented in the form of a workbook and enables local health departments to

- assess and improve their organizational capacity
- assess the health status of their communities
- actively involve their communities in improving public health

For more information and to purchase the workbooks, please contact: APEXPH Manager, NACCHO, 440 First Street NW, Suite 500, Washington, DC 20001. Phone: (202) 783-5550.

■ **Campbell Community Survey**

This survey measures how people feel about the community in which they live, and includes the community aspects of educational programs, environmental protection, healthcare services, housing, safety, serenity, freedom from drugs, and general optimism. Produced to assist communities in identifying strengths and weaknesses, this survey targets those areas of highest concern to community members.

For more information and to purchase the resource, please contact: Paula Vanatta, Center for Creative Leadership, P.O. Box 1559, Colorado Springs, CO 80901. Phone: (719) 633-3891.

■ **Central Oklahoma 2020's Select Community Indicators**

"Central Oklahoma 2020 is a regional, community-based strategic planning process for the four counties and more than 20 municipalities in the Oklahoma City area. . . . Arthur L. Sargent, Executive Director of the Central Oklahoma Community Council, took on the project's primary task of developing a set of quality-of-life indicators for the region. The result, the Central Oklahoma 2020— Select Community Indicators, has become the basis for a series of public presentations and dialogues, and in the future will serve as a standard against which to measure outcomes from community initiatives over the years."

For more information, please contact: Arthur L. Sargent, Executive Director, Community Council of Central Oklahoma, P.O. Box 675, Oklahoma City, OK 73101-0675. Phone: (405) 525-4858. Fax: (405) 525-4852.

■ **Claritas NPDC**

With "Update!," Claritas NPDC presents current-year estimates and five-year projections of demographic data at the community level. Along with Donnelley Marketing Information Services, Claritas offers statistical data in socioeconomic areas, much like the U.S. decennial census, but on a more timely basis.

For more information, please contact: Marketing Department, Claritas NPDC, P.O. Box 610, Ithaca, NY 14851-0610. Phone: (800) 234-5973.

■ **Colorado Healthy Communities Initiative**

The Colorado Healthy Communities Initiative is a five-year effort to establish community-based approaches to address health issues in Colorado. Over the course of the Colorado Healthy Communities Initiative, there are three program cycles, each of which is three years long. Up to thirty communities will be involved over the five-year initiative. The Colorado Healthy Communities Initiative is a project of the Colorado Trust and is managed by the National Civic League.

For information, please contact Julia Weaver, National Civic League, 1445 Market Street, Suite 300, Denver, CO 80202-1728. Phone: (303) 571-4343. Fax: (303) 571-4404.

■ **Community Assessment of Human Needs (second edition, updated 1994)**

The Community Assessment of Human Needs (CAHN) is a systematic approach to identifying and understanding the unmet human needs of populations at risk within the defined community of healthcare providers. The guide is a comprehensive source of information that has been designed to be a flexible tool to provide guidelines and technical assistance. The assessment contains four phases: (1) community characteristics, (2) human service providers, (3) community leaders, and (4) populations at risk. Phase 1 is designed as a quantitative methodology for identifying the populations at risk and where in the community of healthcare providers these populations are most likely located. Phases 2–4 are interactive phases designed with a threefold purpose; they provide an opportunity to validate the data in phase 1 by speaking with people directly informed; they provide vehicles for gathering information (e.g., interview provider, community leaders, and persons at risk), and they create an opportunity to network by identifying needs and discovering new and creative ways to address those needs.

For more information, please contact: Clifford Rowley, Mercy Health Services, 34605 Twelve Mile Road, Farmington Hills, MI 48331. Phone: (810) 489-6759.

■ Community Health Assessment: A Process for Positive Change (1993)

This comprehensive, 182-page book describes how health care organizations can join with the broader community to assess and develop creative, efficient and integrated strategies for addressing local health issues. For healthcare organizations seeking to strengthen their community-focused initiatives, this document offers a detailed description of the community health assessment process. It addresses the strategic fit and conceptual philosophical basis for such an effort, the implementation of a six-phase process, and key challenges and possible solutions that might arise during the various phases.

To order, write to: VHA Community Health Improvement, P.O. Box 14090, Irving, TX 75014-0909 or fax to: (972) 830-0332. Allow four to six weeks for delivery. Please call (800) 842-7587 with ordering questions.

■ The Community Indicators Handbook

The Community Indicators Handbook measures progress toward healthy, sustainable communities. It draws on the experience of dozens of projects around the United States, and presents communities with how-to's and resources for tailoring an indicator project to their specific needs. The handbook is the collaborative product of three organizations: the staff of Tyler Norris Associates, who have worked extensively with dozens of Healthy Cities/Healthy Communities projects; the volunteers of Sustainable Seattle, recognized as both a pioneer and a model program for developing urban sustainability indicators; and the National Indicators Program of Redefining Progress, which is developing a Community Indicators Network to support the spread of these projects nationwide.

This handbook is a joint project of Redefining Progress, Tyler Norris and Associates, and Sustainable Seattle forthcoming in spring-summer 1997 and published by Redefining Progress. For more information, please contact: Kate Besleme at Redefining Progress, 1 Kearny Street, 4th Floor, San Francisco, CA 94108. Phone: (415) 781-1191.

■ Community Services Workstation

A partnership initiative of Howard University School of Social Work and the Health and Human Services Coalition of the District of Columbia, Rice University and Baylor College of Medicine, Marco International, United Seniors Health Cooperative, and Bell Atlantic Corporation, the Community Services Workstation seeks to build an "infrastructure for the coordination of health and human services for families and children." Included in this project is a computerized, integrated workstation that resulted from the development of client profiles; needs assessments; and service eligibility, services brokering and evaluation support tools.

For more information, please contact: Jim Craigen, Howard University School of Social Work, 601 Howard Place NW, Washington, DC 20059. Phone: (202) 806-7324.

■ Community Vitality Index (Gallup, Inc.)

The Community Vitality Index measures a community's quality of life by identifying main themes of different communities. The poll responsible for this index was conducted in fourteen communities where Gallup has an office. The major categories covered in the sixty questions include: leadership, stress/personal health, equity/fairness, diversity, economic/environmental growth, community spirit, and personal support systems.

For more information, please contact: Don Clifton, Gallup, Inc., 301 S. 68th St., Lincoln, NE 68505. Phone: (800) 288-8592.

■ Delaware County's Health Checkup

Delaware County, Pennsylvania, completed an exhaustive community health status assessment under the sponsorship of Crozer-Keystone. The tool was developed with the assistance of the county government, the state health department, the county medical society, healthcare providers and leading local and national healthcare academicians. "This assessment identifies needs and sets priorities for future action. It also establishes very detailed baseline indicators from which to measure progress." Crozer-Keystone learned invaluable lessons from designing this community-specific tool.

For more information, please contact: Ann Bagnell, Marketing Executive, Crozer-Keystone Health System, Rose Tree Corporate Center II, 1400 N. Providence Rd., Suite 4010, Media, PA 19063-2049. Phone: (610) 892-8000. Fax: (610) 892-8030.

■ Donnelley Marketing Information Services

Donnelley Marketing, a company of Dunn and Bradstreet, collects and makes available marketing statistics and information on Standard Metropolitan Statistical Areas in the United States. Their information includes block-level statistics on financial data, retail trade, construction, household mobility and income, population by age, occupied housing by family type, length of residence, etc. Although they do not focus on primary health indicators, Donnelley does provide exhaustive information on the social and economic health indicators of communities.

For more information, please contact: Demographics on Call, 12770 High Bluff Dr., Suite 215, San Diego, CA 92130. Phone: (800) 866-2255.

■ Health Indicator Workbook: A Tool for Healthy Communities (second edition)

This workbook is designed to help communities determine and measure factors that have an impact on individual and community health, including socioeconomic status, social support, and clean and safe physical environments. Designed to help the community develop its own "measures of a healthy community," this source uses both population and community indicators.

For more information, please contact: Don Cumming, Sr. Advisor for Healthier Communities, Office of Health Promotion, British Columbia Ministry of Health and Ministry Responsible for Seniors, 1520 Blanchard Street, First Floor, Victoria, BC V8W 3C8, Canada. Phone: (250) 952-2117.

■ Healthy Futures: A Development Kit for Rural Hospitals

Community Decision Making (CDM) in rural hospital communities is a process that seeks to involve residents of rural communities in developing solutions to problems with local healthcare systems. The project generates citizen participation in rural health public policy decisions. The hospital board of directors endorses the CDM project and hires a community encourager (a local resident) to organize and coordinate the program. CDM has provided background information and techniques to collect different types of data. A very functional tool is a table of data collection methods and a description of how useful the method is in obtaining certain levels of information and of its overall representativeness of the community. Although CDM did not develop specific survey tools, it does provide guidance in the types of information that should be collected, methods for obtaining the information (resources), key questions, interviewing techniques, and other ideas for obtaining community-level data.

For more information, please contact: Paul McGinnis, Mountain States Health Corporation, P.O. Box 6756, Boise, ID 83707. Phone: (208) 342-4666.

■ Hospital Community Benefit Standards Program, New York University

Through a grant from the W. K. Kellogg Foundation, the New York University Robert F. Wagner Graduate School of Public Service developed and field-tested standards for hospitals to help improve community health, address special health problems of the medically underserved, and contain healthcare costs. Forty-nine hospitals and communities participated in this program, which was transitioned to the American Hospital Association in 1992. The AHA will now provide general information on community benefit programs to interested hospitals and health systems, and will be using community benefit programs as a key strategy for the community care network reform initiative.

For more information, please contact: Anthony R. Kovner, PhD, Director, Hospital Community Benefit Standards Program, NYU Wagner Graduate School of Public Service, 600 Tisch Hall, 40 West 4th St., New York, NY 10012. Phone: (212) 998-7444. Fax: (212) 995-4165.

■ Human Development Report and Index

Human Development Report 1990 defined human development as the process of increasing people's options. It stressed that the most critical choices that people should have include the options to lead a long and healthy life, to be knowledgeable, and to find access to the assets, employment, and income needed for a decent standard of living.

Development, thus defined, cannot be adequately measured by income alone. The 1990 report therefore proposed a new measure of development, the human development index (HDI), composed of three indicators: life expectancy, education, and income. For each of the three dimensions, the 1990 report identified minimum achievements worldwide: the lowest national life expectancy, the lowest national level of adult literacy, and the lowest level of income per capita. It also established a maximum or desirable adequate level of attainment.

"Human development cannot take place without human life and health; people do not just want to be alive; they want to know their way around in life. They want to be knowledgeable; and they certainly may want a decent life, one that is not constantly undermined by extreme poverty and the constant worry about sheer physical survival. All three of the HDI components thus deserve equal weight. And that is why the HDI proposes an unweighted average of a country's rank on the life expectancy, literacy, and income scale."

For more information, please contact: Human Development Report Office, United Nations Development Program, 336 East 45th Street, Uganda House, 6th Floor, New York, NY 10017. Phone: (212) 906-3661. Fax: (212) 983-0025.

■ Life in Jacksonville: Quality Indicators for Progress

This study, commissioned by the Jacksonville Chamber of Commerce in 1983, gauges the quality of life in the Jacksonville metropolitan area. "The purpose was to determine indicators that contribute to the community's general feelings of well-being, fulfillment and satisfaction." Seventy-four indicators are identified in this annual study, providing important longitudinal data that allow citizens to set quality-of-life targets for the year 2000.

For more information, please contact: Anna Scheu, Vice President of Business, Jacksonville Chamber of Commerce, 3 Independent Drive, Jacksonville, FL Phone: (904) 366-6650. Fax: (904) 632-0617.

■ Minnesota Department of Public Health, Community Health Promotion Kit

This kit is a manual that contains a collection of resources, tip sheets, activities, and technical assistance tools that have been developed and used by communities across the United States. Key features of the program include data assessment and coalition building strategies, program design, and techniques on how to involve the media. Section 1 of the manual is devoted to determining the health of the community by using federal, state and local data resources.

For more information, please contact: Karen McComas, Health Director, Minnesota Department of Health, 717 Delaware Street, SE, Minneapolis, MN 55440-9441. Phone: (612) 623-5000.

■ National Center for Health Statistics

As part of the Department of Health and Human Services, the National Center for Health Statistics publishes results of such surveys as the National Health Interview Survey, the National Health and Examination Survey, the Hospital Discharge Survey, and the National Ambulatory Medical Care Survey, among other publications that list morbidity and mortality statistics, and other vital statistics. Although some information is community-specific, this government agency also provides an excellent national health picture that individual communities can use as a comparison to their own health status.

For more information, please contact: U.S. Department of Health and Human Services, Public Health Service, Centers for Disease Control, National Center for

Health Statistics, 3700 East-West Highway, Hyattsville, MD 20782.
Phone: (301) 436-8500.

■ **National Civic League: The Civic Index**

Developed as a way to evaluate communities' civic infrastructure, this index provides methods for identifying a community's strengths and weaknesses as well as collaborative problem-solving techniques. There are ten components of the index that correlate to specific skills needed to address community problems.

For more information, please contact: National Civic League, 1445 Market St., Suite 300, Denver, CO 80202-1728. Phone: (303) 571-4343. Fax: (303) 571-4404.

■ **Pasadena's Quality of Life Index**

Developed for the City of Pasadena, California, and from Pasadena's own Healthy Cities Project, this index can be used as a helpful tool for other communities that wish to develop their own quality of life scale. The index includes eleven key areas, ranging from the arts to health and the environment. Particularly useful in monitoring progress toward healthier community goals, this tool is an excellent benchmark.

For more information, please contact: Deborah L. Silver, Healthy Cities Project Manager, City of Pasadena, 100 North Garfield Avenue, Room 136, Pasadena, CA 91109. Phone: (818) 844-6050.

■ **Planned Approach to Community Health (PATCH)**

Designed to help communities plan, implement and evaluate health promotion and health education programs, PATCH is a process through which partners address the healthcare needs of the community. PATCH partners include the Centers for Disease Control, the state health department, and the community. The program consists of six workshops in which participating community members gain skills in five key areas of community health promotion: community organization, data collection, establishing priorities and setting objectives, intervention planning, and evaluation. Currently seventeen states and fifty communities have initiated PATCH programs.

For more information, please contact: Nancy B. Watkins, Division of Chronic Disease Control and Community Intervention, Centers for Disease Control, 1600 Clifton Rd., N.E., Mailstop K-46, Atlanta, GA 30333. Phone: (770) 488-5435.

■ **Snohomish County Needs Assessment Project, Snohomish County, Washington**

"Begun in 1989 and updated periodically (last done in 1995), the Snohomish County Needs Assessment Project is a joint effort of the United Way of Snohomish County, the Snohomish County Department of Health and Human Services, and the Everett/Snohomish County Impact Coordinating Council. The purpose of the project is to establish priorities for health and human needs in Snohomish County and to develop a plan to direct community resources to meet those needs. The assessment process was based on the United Way's community needs assessment program, COMPASS."

The project was directed by a steering committee consisting of approximately thirty community leaders who represent a wide range of perspectives about the community. The survey information was gathered by a professional research firm directed by a separate survey committee. Social and economic indicators were collected by a separate data collection committee.

For more information, please contact: Dean Hanks, President, United Way of Snohomish County, 917 134th Street S.W., Suite A-6, Everett, WA 98204. Phone: (206) 742-5911. Fax: (206) 743-1440.

■ Somerville Hospital and Somerville Health Department

Using APEXPH, Somerville conducted an exhaustive "current health status" of its community, developing and distributing its health assessment survey to three hundred community leaders and one hundred health providers. This survey represents a unique, community-specific marriage of a standard assessment tool and a local survey.

For more information, please contact: Linda M. Cundiff, Vice President of Community Health Services, Somerville Hospital, 230 Highland Ave., Somerville, MA 02143. Phone: (617) 666-4400. Fax: (617) 666-0031.

■ Stanford Health Promotion Resource Center, Health Promotion in Diverse Cultural Communities

The manual for this program focuses on techniques and strategies designed to aid the "health educator" in the access, design, and implementation of a health promotion program within a diverse cultural community. Specific techniques for conducting a needs assessment are presented.

For more information, please contact: Health Promotion Resource Center, Stanford University, 1000 Welch Road, Palo Alto, CA 94304-1885. Phone: (415) 723-0003.

■ SF-36 Health Status Questionnaire (1993)

Based on Medical Outcomes Study (MOS) surveys, this questionnaire was developed in 1993 to measure health and evaluate generic health concepts. Meant to be used as part of a larger outcomes management system, this tool is easy to administer and takes only a few minutes to complete, while maintaining reliability and validity.

For more info and to purchase the survey, please contact: Health Outcomes Institute, 2001 Killebrew Dr., Suite 122, Bloomington, MN 55425. Phone: (612) 858-9188. Fax: (612) 858-9189.

■ State Data Centers

In conjunction with the U.S. Bureau of the Census, many states have established data centers that make census information available and assist state and local governments and community, business, and private organizations in interpreting census materials. Among their services are community and census tract statistics in the areas of population and housing, including socioeconomic data, population projections, and mortality statistics.

For the name, address and phone number of the state data center nearest you, please contact: U.S. Bureau of the Census, State Data Center Information, at (301) 457-1713.

■ **The Sustainable Seattle: Indicators of Sustainable Community**

"These proposed 'Indicators of Sustainable Community' are the product of a creative community dialogue about our common future. . . . This array of indicators is intended to provide a snapshot of the concept of sustainability. . . . Indicators are bits of information that reflect the status of large systems. They are a way of seeing the 'big picture' by looking at a smaller piece of it. They tell us which direction a system is going: up or down, forward or backward, getting better or worse or staying the same."

For more information, please contact: Sustainable Seattle, c/o Metrocenter YMCA, 909 4th Avenue, Seattle, WA 98103. Phone: (206) 382-5013.

■ **United Way of America (COMPASS)**

"COMPASS is a comprehensive guide which will assist any community. It is a tool that enables local communities to learn about local needs (all needs, or a specific issue or target group) and to develop and implement a community action plan. . . . Three kinds of survey questionnaires are included in both brief and in-depth versions. Software is included which can be used on any IBM-compatible computer for tabulating survey results. Further, COMPASS includes worksheets for organizing the social and economic data that is analyzed."

For more information, please contact Curt Johnson, Director, Community Problem Solving, United Way of America, 701 North Fairfax St., Alexandria, VA 22314-2045. Phone: (703) 836-7100.

■ **U.S. Bureau of the Census**

The U.S. Bureau of the Census, Department of Commerce, conducts the decennial census of housing and population as well as various five-year censuses of retail, manufacturing and service industries. They also conduct regular population surveys of most urban areas. They are a rich source for census tract and block statistics of education, income, occupation, size of families, housing (including single- and multi-family dwellings), language spoken at home, and many other socioeconomic indicators. With more than fourteen hundred federal depository libraries housing these materials, most communities have ready access to this wealth of information. State and local governments may also publish statistics and materials of interest to your community.

For information on the depository library nearest you, please contact your local public library.

■ **Washington State Hospital Association, 1992 Community and Hospital Issues and Priorities Survey**

Administered to government and community leaders, this survey assessed "priorities civic and community leaders place on a wide range of local concerns, including those affecting health care." It evaluated community needs, views of hospitals' performance on healthcare issues and community issues, perceptions about hospitals, awareness of hospitals' performance, future importance of hospital resources, and other areas. An excellent source for ideas when creating your own survey or questionnaire, this survey presents an exhaustive list of questions.

For more information, please contact: Leslie Thorpe, Public Relations Director, Public Affairs, Washington State Hospital Association, 190 Queen Anne Avenue North, Third Floor, Seattle, WA 98109. Phone: (206) 281-7211.

Collaboration and Coalition Building

■ **Building Communities from the Inside Out: A Path Toward Finding and Mobilizing a Community's Assets, by John Kretzmann and John McKnight**

John McKnight's writing has been an inspiration to coalition builders and community developers for many years. This newest addition to the McKnight library is outstanding. Up to this point, McKnight has been an insightful critic of what is wrong with the health and human service system. In *Building Communities from the Inside Out*, Kretzmann and McKnight lay out a clear, step-by-step process for doing asset assessment to increase individual capacities and to release the power of local associations and organizations. They go on to describe how to capture local institutions for community building, and break that down by parks, schools, libraries, community colleges, hospitals, etc. Finally, the remainder of the book focuses on rebuilding a community economy. While you're at it, check out the rest of the publications from the Center for Urban Affairs and Policy Research, including: *Mapping Community Capacity*, an earlier version of *Building Communities from the Inside Out*. Available by writing to: Center for Urban Affairs and Policy Research, Northwestern University, 2040 Sheridan Road, Evanston, IL 60208-4100. Phone: (708) 491-8712. Fax: (708) 491-9916. ($12.00 p.pd.)

■ **Coalition for Healthy Cities and Communities in the United States**

This coalition is an excellent resource for communities looking for guidance on their Healthier Community initiatives. The objective of the coalition is to communicate the vision, mission and goals of the Coalition for Healthy Cities and Communities in the United States and the principles of the Healthy Community movement to a broad range of audiences and diverse community systems. The goal is to increase awareness and the number of Healthy Community efforts by providing information and assistance to support their initiation and development. Additional information is available by contacting: Hospital Research and Education Trust, One North Franklin, Chicago, IL 60606. Phone: (312) 422-2624.

■ **Coalition Building: One Path to Empowered Communities (1991)**

This 37-page paper, written by Tom Wolff, PhD, is based on eight years of coalition-building experience in Massachusetts. It highlights characteristics of dysfunctional helping systems (fragmentation, duplication of effort, competition, multicultural insensitivity, etc.), characteristics of competent helping systems (coordination, cooperation, cultural relevance, etc.) and the coalition-building strategies needed to move toward greater competence. The paper lays the groundwork for the purpose and direction of coalition building. The author defines healthy and competent communities as the ultimate goals of coalition building and community development activities. Case studies, drawn from the author's direct experiences, give examples of how coalitions can succeed. Available for $10.00 from Community Partners, 24 South Prospect Street, Amherst, MA 01002.

■ **The Community Collaboration Manual, by the National Assembly of National Voluntary Health and Social Welfare Organizations (1991)**

This 76-page manual is extremely well written, and very clear, with many helpful tables and figures. It leads the reader through the process of collaboration, defining collaboration, talking about start-up, building the collaboration, maintaining the momentum, youth involvement, business involvement, and the role of the media. An example of this manual's helpful tips include their seven keys to successful collaboration: shared vision, skilled leadership, process orientation, cultural diversity, membership-driven agenda, multiple sectors, and accountability. Although somewhat more expensive ($12.95), it is packed with good ideas and good models. It is extremely helpful. To order a copy, make check payable to "The National Assembly," and write to: Collaboration Manual, the National Assembly, 1319 F Street NW, Suite 601, Washington, DC 20004.

■ **Community Development, Community Participation and Substance Abuse Prevention, by David Chavis and Paul Florin (May 1990)**

This 25-page pamphlet, developed for the Prevention Office of Drug Abuse Services in San Jose, California, lays out the theoretical understanding behind community development and community participation as they relate to substance abuse prevention. Chavis and Florin define the key concepts regarding community development, and then indicate the key reasons why the community development approach to substance abuse can be especially helpful. These two short papers provide a key rationale and set of definitions for those developing substance abuse prevention coalitions. This is a must-read for substance abuse coalitions. "Community Development, Community Participation and Substance Abuse Prevention" ($5.00 p.pd.) is available from the Bureau of Drug Abuse Services, 645 South Bascom Ave., Building H-10, San Jose, CA 95128.

■ **Community Partnerships: Taking Charge of Change Through Partnership (1993)**

This 56-page document examines partnerships that address a particular community health problem or develop a broad-based, community-wide coalition based on a shared vision for community health. It includes a bibliography as well as profiles of health improvement projects and programs that have succeeded because of community partnerships.

To order, write to: VHA Community Health Improvement, P.O. Box 14090, Irving, TX, 75014-0909, or fax to: (972) 830-0332. Allow four to six weeks for delivery. Please call (800) 842-7587 with ordering questions.

■ **Communities Working Collaboratively for a Change, by Arthur Turovh Himmelman (July 1992 edition)**

Himmelman does an outstanding job of defining collaboration and distinguishing it from networking, coordination and cooperation. He describes two kinds of multisectoral collaboration—collaborative betterment and collaborative empowerment—and articulates both in a very helpful model. He then goes on to describe his own model for collaborative empowerment. Excellent, thought-provoking paper from a citizen participation–government perspective. Cost for this monograph is $10.00 p.pd. To order, please contact: the Himmelman Consulting Group, 1406 West Lake Street, Suite 209, Minneapolis, MN 55408.

■ **The Foundation Center's Fundraising and Nonprofit Development Resources (Summer 1996)**

The Foundation Center is an independent nonprofit organization whose mission is to increase public understanding of foundations. They accomplish this by maintaining a comprehensive and up-to-date database on foundations and corporate giving programs, by producing directories, and by analyzing trends in foundation support of the nonprofit sector. For more information, please contact: the Foundation Center, 79 Fifth Avenue/16th Street, New York, NY 10003-3076. Phone (800) 424-9836.

■ **Organizing for Social Change, by Kim Bobo, Jackie Kendall, and Steve Max**

This is a manual for activists in the 1990s, and it comes out of the Midwest Academy, one of the most prestigious organizing training centers in the country. This is focused less on coalition building and more on direct action, organizing, organizing skills, and the steps involved in becoming a good organizer. A well written, clear and especially helpful manual. Seven Locks Press, P.O. Box 27, Cabin John, MD 20818. $19.95 plus $2 shipping.

■ **Partnerships for Community Development, by Sally Habana Hafner and Horace Reed**

This excellent publication out of the Center for Organizational and Community Development of the University of Massachusetts-Amherst (an organization that followed the Citizen Involvement Training Project, whose publications were also excellent) provides a wonderful overview of partnership behavior and partnerships in general. They carefully distinguish various types of partnerships, including networks, coordination and collaboration. Especially helpful are the many exercises for groups to use as they go through the text. It is available from the Center for Organizational and Community Development, 377 Hills South, University of Massachusetts, Amherst, MA 01003 ($15.00 plus $2.50 shipping, bulk discount available).

■ **Resources from The Work Group on Health Promotion and Community Development, by Steve Fawcett, Adrienne Paine-Andrews, and Vince Francisco**

The Work Group on Health Promotion and Community Development is producing some of the best materials for coalition building in the country, including: *Preventing Substance Abuse: An Action Planning Guide for Community-Based Initiatives* and *Preventing Adolescent Pregnancy: An Action Planning Guide for Community-Based Initiatives.* These are excellent step-by-step guides that take a coalition through the planning stages, including identifying community changes in each sector of the community. Superb manuals, $12 each, p.pd. *Evaluation Handbook: Evaluating and Supporting Initiatives for Community Health and Development* begins with an overview of The Work Group's system for successfully evaluating community health initiatives, including coalitions. Each measurement instrument, its form and instructions, are explained and sampled, and sample data is given in a presentation form (graphs or summary reports).

Blank forms are included. ($25, p.pd.) Write to: The Work Group, University of Kansas, 4001 Dole Building, Lawrence, KS, 66045.

■ **Solving Community Problems by Consensus; Facing Racial and Cultural Conflict; and Involving Citizens in Community Decision Making**

These are three excellent manuals, all developed by a remarkable man with a remarkable organization—Bill Potachuck and the Program for Community Problem Solving in Washington, DC. They have been developing materials and programs to help communities solve problems for many years. These are excellent and usable manuals and in addition to these titles, there are three volumes of case studies, featuring successful community problem solving; the national directory of problem-solving consultants; and a bibliography on building communities. Each of these is attractively designed and well organized, with no-nonsense advice and detailed resource lists. For a complete description of materials and prices, please contact: the Program for Community Problem Solving, 915 15th Street, NW, 6th Floor, Washington, DC 20005. Phone: (202) 783-2961.

■ **Washington Health Foundation's Community Health Resource Center**

A tremendous boon for anyone attempting to make a significant difference in his or her community, the Washington Health Foundation's Community Health Resource Center provides information on successful health improvement efforts from all over the country. Detailed information is available on a vast array of projects, including teen pregnancy prevention, youth literacy, violence prevention, programs for older adults, and more. The Center provides summary descriptions for each program as well as in-depth analysis and auxiliary materials (such as journal articles and videotapes) where available. An outstanding source of ideas and shared lessons from innovative programs throughout the nation.

To explore the Resource Center online, set your Internet browser to www.whf.org, or contact Linda Klein, Washington Health Foundation, 300 Elliott Ave. W., Suite 300, Seattle, Washington, 98119-4118 (lindak@wha.org). Phone: (800) 226-0720

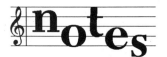

Overhead Slides

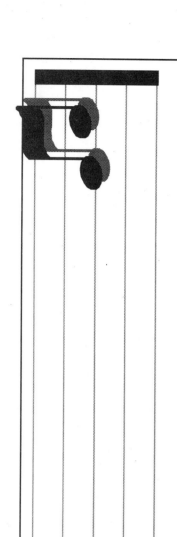

Best Practices in Collaboration to Improve Health

Creating Community Jazz

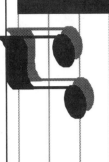

Organizing the Effort

- Agree on mission, values, and principles of the effort
- Agree on a process for working together
- Design organizational structure
- Determine meeting guidelines
- Define roles and responsibilities

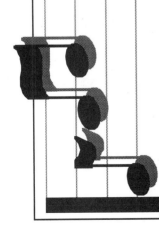

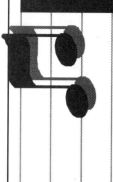

Organizing
the Effort (cont.)

- Create an effective process for communication

- Coordinate budget and fund development

- Link with other efforts

- Celebrate!

- Promote the effort

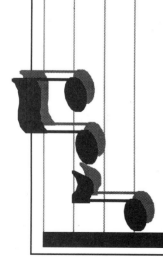

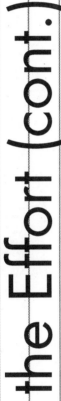

Organizing the Effort (cont.)

- Build the leadership capacity of all stakeholders

- Enlist technical assistance and support

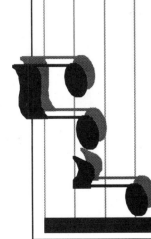

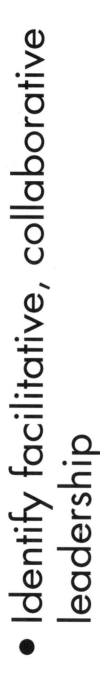

Convening the Community

- Identify facilitative, collaborative leadership
- Define the scope and parameters of the effort
- Develop and implement effective vehicles for two-way communication
- Research potential stakeholders

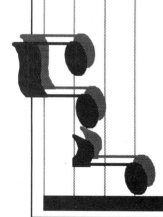

© The Healthcare Forum

Convening the Community (cont.)

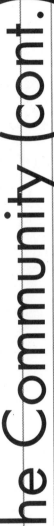

- Invite stakeholders
- Build trust and credibility within the stakeholder community

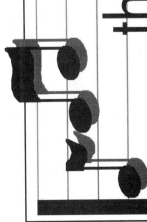

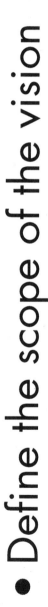

Creating
a Shared Vision

- Define the scope of the vision

- Design the visioning event

- Conduct the visioning event

- Follow up

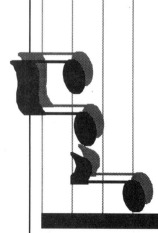

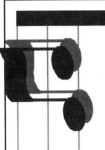

Assessing Current Realities and Trends

- Determine who conducts the assessment, and when

- Frame the assessment process

- Collect secondary data

- Map assets

- Consider primary data

- Inform the public

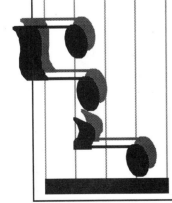

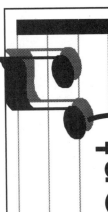

Assessing Current Realities and Trends (cont.)

- Collect primary data
- Validate and benchmark
- Prioritize
- Report findings

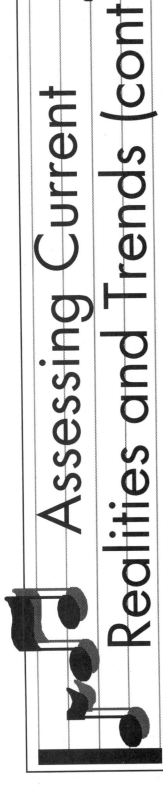

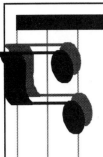

Action Planning

- Define the purpose of an action plan
- Develop a framework
- Conduct design meetings to create the action plan
- Write the initial action plan
- Validate and revise the action plan
- Disseminate the action plan

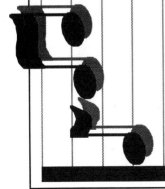

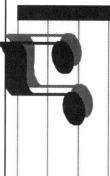

Doing the Job

- Capitalize on strengths
- Find more partners
- Get buy-in
- Get and maintain resources
- Get the word out
- Undertake projects and initiatives
- Deliver the "goods"

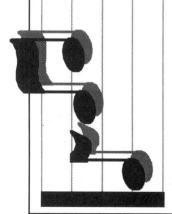

© The Healthcare Forum

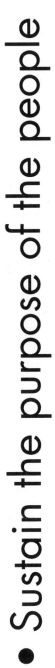

Doing the Job (cont.)

- Sustain the purpose of the people

- Stay focused and fine-tune

Monitoring and Adjusting

- Develop shared ideas and values for a monitoring system
- Clarify goals and objectives
- Develop measures, tools and indicators
- Develop evaluation design
- Collect data
- Synthesize and analyze data

Monitoring and Adjusting (cont.)

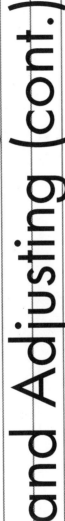

- Report results, findings and feedback

- Recognize successes and challenges

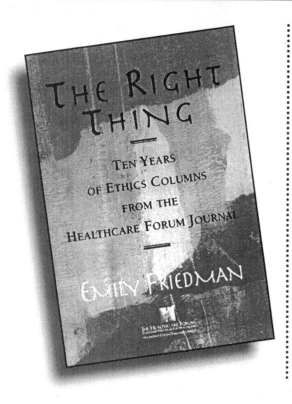
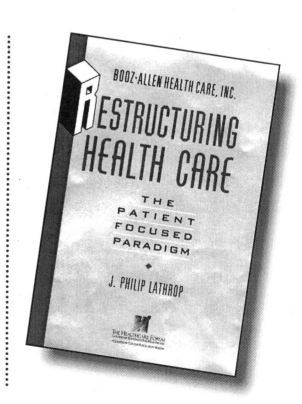